Breastfeeding and the Working Mother

Breastfeeding and the Working Mother

REVISED EDITION

DIANE MASON and
DIANE INGERSOLL

with an Introduction by
Kittie Frantz, R.N., C.P.N.P.

St. Martin's Griffin 🐾 New York

Library of Congress Cataloging-in-Publication Data

Mason, Diane.
    Breastfeeding and the working mother / by Diane Mason and Diane
Ingersoll ; with an introduction by Kittie Frantz.—Rev. ed.
        p. cm.
    Includes bibliographical references.
    ISBN 0-312-15486-0
    1. Breast feeding.   2. Working mothers.   I. Ingersoll, Diane.
II. Title.
RJ216.M37   1997
649'.33—dc21   97-2329
                                                                         CIP

First St. Martin's Griffin Edition: July 1997   5|17|99

10   9   8   7   6   5   4   3   2   1

For my sister, Susan—I breastfed because she did.
And for Ann and Tom—the ones I breastfed.

—DM

For Eric, my son, and Hilary, my daughter—
they inspired me;
Paul, my husband—your support was invaluable;
and for Mom and Dad—who taught me endurance.

—DI

Contents

Acknowledgments

Special thanks to:

Sarah Danner, Certified Pediatric Nurse Practitioner and Certified Nurse Midwife in Peterborough, New Hampshire, and member of executive board of the U.S. Baby Friendly Hospital Initiative.

Diane L. Dimperio, M.A., R.D., Associate in Obstetrics and Gynecology, University of Florida, College of Medicine, Gainesville, Florida.

Patricia M. Lee, Attorney at Law, 572 1st Avenue North, St. Petersburg, Florida 33701

Ronald G. Meyer, Esquire, Meyer and Brooks, 2544 Blairstone Pines Drive, Tallahassee, Florida 32301.

David L. Peterman, M.D., and the staff of Pediatric Associates of Boise, Idaho.

The staff of the Idaho State Law Library.

The staff of Idaho WIC Program.

Our agent, Susan Ann Protter.

Nancy Rosenheim, Karen Barnard, Kris Hudson, Lynn Wilson, Susan Ingersoll, Linda Blackman, Kathleen Auerback, Abby J. Cohen, Howard and Denise Carsman, Ridley Pearson, Pam Lodal, Richard Skinner, Joanne Graff, Debbie Kannenberg, Sharon Bixby, Linda Morton, Dave Flynn, and Donna R. McBride.

And a special, heartfelt thanks to all of the women we interviewed, whose experiences, and their willingness to share them, made this book possible.

Introduction

As a young mother I'd climb our apartment stairs after a day at work and hear my eight-month-old son's eager anticipation. "Ah-huh, ah-huh, ah-huh," he exclaimed as he bounced up and down in his flexible seat, hearing my footsteps on the stairs. This used to unnerve the babysitter who would protest that he had been just fine all day. She viewed his eagerness to see me and his immediate desire to nurse as a reproach to her care. She had fed him well all day so why did he act as if he were starving when I came home?

Settling into a chair to nurse my son after a hard day's work made everything right again. A sense of peace would flood over me. It was as if my feet touched the ground in one stroke of reality. That was what life was really about then. My children, my babies were my focus—the job a mere necessity. Nursing after a hard day of work put it all into perspective. I felt very fulfilled and at peace as my two-year-old climbed up onto the couch to snuggle and hear a story as I nursed the baby. Dinner would be late again.

This was the early 1960s when few women worked if they

had young children and fewer still actually breastfed their babies, even if they stayed home. My husband was finishing school at UCLA and the job market was tight, so we had no choice.

At that time, there were no readily available electric breast pumps to rent and only two hand breast pumps on the market. I didn't pump at work, as I had no one to advise me. I was lucky however, and worked for a German obstetrician, Dorothea Behne, who simply said, "Just nurse when you are home. That's what I did. The trick is to nurse a lot on your days off to rebuild your supply." She was very supportive in our workplace and my baby weaned himself at one year of age. Today's working mother has many more helpful choices. Nowadays there are 173 products on the market for the breast-feeding mother. Chapter Four in the book highlights a few that are helpful for a working woman who plans to breastfeed.

Workplaces are becoming "breastfeeding friendly" as large corporations develop lactation programs to assist and encourage their employees to breastfeed. The most valuable part of this book is Chapter Eleven, "Your Legal Right to Breast-feed." Women who find their workplace inflexible with their plans to return to work and breastfeed will learn new ways to negotiate. There is a lot of power in being a valuable employee, and remember—it may be more expensive to replace you.

As fate would have it, I didn't begin to work until little John was several months old. I didn't know it then, but this may have been why I was able to work and breastfeed so successfully.

Cultures all over the world have ancient rules about the first thirty to forty days after the baby is born. These rules center on the confinement of mother and infant. In Latin America it is called *cuarentena,* which means "forty" to reflect the forty days or six weeks that mother and baby stay at home. In China it is *zuo yué haizi,* literally "sit-month-child," and encompasses one complete moon cycle or thirty days that mother and baby should be confined at home. These confinement periods are found in Africa, Asia, and the Americas.

Why confined? There is nothing wrong with childbirth.

The mother wasn't sick. The feminist hairs on the back of my neck used to rise as I heard my Latina patients and foreign-born medical students speak of this in the 1980s. But the more I inquired about the "rules" for this period of confinement, the more I saw wisdom in it. I even envied the pampering of the mother and newly delivered child that our culture seems to have abandoned. The women around the new mother cook for the family, do laundry and market, and care for the other children. The mother and baby are always kept warm, especially the mother's breasts, and ritual foods and herbs are prepared for her. She is truly a queen with nothing to do but nurse her infant.

After I settled back down from my awe, I studied the physiology of lactation and learned that the level of the milk-making hormone, prolactin, is very high in a woman's blood during the first six weeks (forty days) after delivery. This hormone gradually decreases after that. How, then, do some woman sustain a milk supply for one, two, or three years? I pondered. Could it be that the six weeks of high prolactin levels, created solely by breastfeeding during that confinement time, produced a reaction in the breast, making the breast self-sustaining later? Was there some kind of receptor site in the breast? Did ancient people around the globe discover that if they kept mother and baby together for these thirty to forty days that the infant's chance of survival improved? In other words, the infants survived when the milk supply was "set" by keeping the woman out of the village work duties for this confinement period. The frequent nursing would keep the levels of the milk-making hormone, prolactin, high in her blood. Was this why I was able to nurse my son as long as I did? Baby John and I were home for the first several months, and I had no plans to return to work, so I just nursed him. We didn't need bottles at all during this period at home. Had I inadvertantly "set" my milk supply, allowing me to go to work later and easily sustain it?

Working mothers are not new to humanity by any means. Women have worked, their infants on their backs, in fields planting rice, gathering nuts and berries, tending goats, and so on. Only the separation of mother and baby that usually occurs when the modern woman returns to work is new.

I worked as a pediatric nurse practitioner and as my knowledge evolved, I began to suggest that my patients use their six-week maternity leave with their infants to "set" the milk supply by nursing. Pumping was begun at two weeks, but that milk was stored and not given to the baby until Mom returned to work. This has been a phenomenal success for my patients. The occasional baby who refused the bottle was easily and temporarily fed by cup by the sitter.

Take seriously the parts in chapters five and nine that discuss how to negotiate help. Today, the village women have to be "hired" in the form of a cleaning person, nanny, personal assistant, and so on. I urge you to consider hiring help if you can afford it so you can enjoy your family or your days off. And treat your maternity leave as a sabbatical to rest and enjoy your baby and family. It can be truly a milk-building time as well as a bond-building one. Don't take "confinement" too literally. Why not take baby with you on family outings?

Breastfeeding and the Working Mother will guide you in planning for and nursing your baby when you return to work. It is with envy that I view the suggestions you will get in this book, for there weren't many for me. Two things I will whisper to you as you embark on this wonderful endeavor to give your baby the best. One is: honour *cuarentena* and pamper yourself while you "set" your milk supply during your maternity leave. The second is the advice from Dorothea that was so simple then—just nurse your baby a lot when you are home (on your days off).

Oh yes, baby John grew to manhood and his wife nursed their first son for eleven months while working full time. Dorothea, who delivered John, must be smiling.

—*Kittie Frantz, R.N., C.P.N.P.*
Director, Breastfeeding Infant Clinic,
Los Angeles County University of
Southern California, Medical Center

Preface

Fifteen years ago, when I was pregnant with Eric, I read everything I could get my hands on about pregnancy, birth, and baby care.

Everything I could find, that is.

There were plenty of materials on breastfeeding, but not one good book about working and breastfeeding. And I was planning to go back to my job as a full-time property manager when my maternity leave ended. I was desperate for some ideas and helpful hints.

I went to several classes on breastfeeding, but none of them addressed the working/breastfeeding mother. It was as if you weren't supposed to do both at the same time!

So I struggled along, on my own and with the support of my husband and a handful of friends. But it bothered me that there was such a gap here. Certainly there were other women who wanted to keep breastfeeding when they went back to work—women who could use some help, not to mention encouragement. I decided to write the book I never could find.

It might be too late to answer my own questions, but I can at least help other mothers with theirs.

It seemed to me that there should be one book that told it all—everything from breastfeeding basics to day care to legal issues in the workplace. The working mother doesn't have time to read a stack of books on the subject, nor does she have time to wade through a tome. The book I envisioned would hit all of the important questions about breastfeeding, offer lots of practical advice and experiences from interviews with other working/breastfeeding mothers, and be short and to the point.

This book is not meant to make you feel guilty if working and breastfeeding doesn't finally suit you. It's not meant to pressure you into working and breastfeeding in the first place. We just want to provide enough information for you to make an informed decision, the one that is best for you and your baby.

Three years after the publication of the first edition of this book, my daughter Hilary was born. Breastfeeding her, I not only benefitted from my own experience, but also from the combined experience of the many women who contributed to this book. Life was a lot easier. So in this second edition, we bring even more to the working/breastfeeding story. I hope this book will make your path a bit easier and your baby happy and healthy.

—Diane Ingersoll

When Diane Ingersoll first approached me with the idea of collaborating on a book about working and breastfeeding, my first reaction was: Work and breastfeed at the same time? Women do that?

When I breastfed my babies (now 21 and 23!), it was all I could do to keep up with the house, baby care, and what seemed like a frenetic family life. I couldn't imagine having a full-time or even a part-time job on top of that. I had left a banking career to start a family, and frankly, at that time there was little support for women in the workplace—let alone a woman who might try to blend a profession and a family. It was naturally assumed that when I left my job to become pregnant, that was the last anyone would see of me for a long time.

In those days, too, there was much less encouragement to breastfeed. And for me, breastfeeding did not come naturally. Oh, there were some nurses who helped out when I put my first baby, Ann, to the breast, but mostly they told me to watch the clock and warned me not to exceed three minutes per side. If it hadn't been for my sister, a husband who reread Karen Pryor's book *Nursing Your Baby* as often as I did, and a new parent support group, I doubt that Ann (and Tom two years later) would have been breastfed babies. As it turned out, both of them were weaned right from the breast to the cup and peanut butter sandwiches.

You can imagine how I felt when Diane told me there were lots of women who breastfeed and work (or want to). I wondered: What kind of woman can take on so much at one time? How does she do it?

Diane told me she had breastfed and worked full time for seventeen months. And my most striking impression of her at first was that she is so easygoing. She isn't frantic, overloaded, or, to use the pop phrase, stressed-out. She seems peaceful and calm and in control of her life. She has a great sense of humor and an even stronger desire to help other women.

As we began researching the book and talking with other women who were working and breastfeeding, I encountered those qualities again and again. I developed a tremendous admiration for these mothers, who were doing what did not even seem like an option to me twenty years ago. What struck me most was that these women are not supermothers. To them, "having it all" is not something reserved for glossy overachievers on the covers of magazines.

Women who work and breastfeed don't think of themselves as doing the impossible. And they don't see themselves as people who are trying to have it all. To want to work and breastfeed your baby is *not* asking too much. It is a natural and reasonable choice, and a fair expectation for any woman to have.

That's what I learned from writing this book—and that's what I hope we can share with you.

Another thing I remember from my breastfeeding days is that I was (and still am) one of those people who are often intimidated by what I read. While I pored relentlessly over parenting books, I frequently felt guilty if I wasn't doing what the book said to do, or if, heaven forbid, I encountered someone who was doing "more" than I was.

Our book is not meant to make you feel guilty if this is not the path for you. It is not meant to persuade you to work and breastfeed. You may or may not decide to continue breastfeeding when you go back to work, but we do hope this book will help you to make an informed decision, and most of all, offer you friendship and support for whatever choice you make.

Our book does not have all the answers. But it does have the latest information on how to breastfeed, and how to breastfeed and work. It has been reviewed by lactation experts, and all of the practical ideas and tips we suggest have come from those who know best. We went directly to the source—working/breastfeeding mothers—and found out.

The first edition of this book was published ten years ago. The copy you are holding is the second edition, something we never in our wildest dreams expected to write. Why? Because we thought that surely within the next decade, the attitudes and atmosphere of our nation's workplaces would shift to accommodate working/breastfeeding mothers fully. We thought our book would be obsolete, not needed in a new, enlightened work world.

That has not been the case. Progress? Yes. But while many employers have acted on behalf of breastfeeding mothers and their families, many have not, and change has been slow. The premise of this book is still viable, and the information still much needed.

I still hope someday this book becomes obsolete. I hope that soon there will be so much support and concern built into the fabric of our whole business system that there will be no such thing as making a *choice* between family and job—that the terms *balancing act* and *juggling* will be anachronisms, and all of us, men and women alike, will be able to put the needs of our families first, freely and openly, with the full backing of the places where we work.

—Diane Mason

Breastfeeding and the Working Mother

Why Breastfeed?

"The doctor put her right up on me. I nursed her within the first ten minutes, and she took right to it. It was one of the first things I wanted to do, and I don't even know why, because I hadn't really researched it or read articles or anything. It was just something—I don't know why I wanted to try it— I just thought, well, here she comes into the world and it was breakfast time and I wanted to nurse her. So I gave it a try."

In that inimitable way she has of knowing exactly what we need, nature has devised a near-perfect way for us to feed our babies. From the beginning of your pregnancy your body has been making preparations, so that by the time you give birth you are fully equipped to provide the best food your baby can get.

Luckily, your baby comes into the world with an instinct for just what to do. She knows how to suckle and has probably been practicing on her own little fist for some time. She also has a *rooting reflex*—when you touch her cheek she will turn her head and open and close her mouth in search of a nipple. And if she is like many alert newborns, she will be ready to go the moment you take her in your arms. Although her vision is limited at first, she can focus about eight inches, not coincidentally the approximate distance from her eyes to yours when she is nursing. Wide-eyed and curious, she will regard you intently as she latches on to the nipple, and her sucking will stimulate your body to release prolactin and oxytocin, the two hormones responsible for lactation. As she nestles against you, your skin provides essential warmth and protection against heat loss after birth. She feels safe. With amazing synchronism, the two of you will set into motion the source of her nourishment—and the beginnings of a very special bond.

From a mother's point of view, how instinctive is breastfeeding? We know it is for most animals, but in the case of people (and some higher primates, such as chimpanzees and gorillas) breastfeeding is also influenced by learning and by imitation of other females. Back when babies were born at home, before birth became the medical and increasingly technological happening it is today, a mother was more apt to automatically put her newborn baby to her breast immediately after birth. However, she did so partly because this is what all the other mothers did, because she grew up observing babies at the breast, and because this was simply the way babies were fed. Today, hospital procedures are not always conducive to a spontaneous birth-to-breast encounter. Also, many women in this generation did not have mothers who breastfed. If you have had few opportunities to observe other women breastfeeding, you may feel awkward or unsure of how to do it. Although breastfeeding is easy and convenient, it does not always come completely naturally. In fact, most mothers today find that success with breastfeeding is best assured when they have a lot of knowledge, information, and support before they begin.

BREASTFEEDING: THEN AND NOW

Like childbirth, and in fact most other aspects of our health care, breastfeeding has become methodological, the object of a great deal of scientific observation and study. The good news is that as our pool of medical knowledge increases, so do the number of healthy babies. The more we understand how our bodies function and, most important, how our babies grow and thrive, the better our chances of providing the optimum environment for their health and well-being. Yet as breastfeeding becomes less an art handed down from generation to generation and more a science, we feel alienated from our own intuitive knowledge. We begin to believe things are much more complicated than they really are and wonder: If women have been breastfeeding for millennia without the benefit of books and statistics, why do we need all this extra help to get off to a good start? Why, for example, should we read this book?

Certainly, one answer to this question is, ironically, progress. Prior to the Industrial Revolution, breastfeeding was a matter of course, unquestioned and economically necessary. Then, enter technology. Our lives became mechanized and urbanized, and our life-styles changed dramatically. Women found it economically necessary to work in factories, a type of work at that time that was not at all compatible with the care and feeding of infants. At the same time, science was making all kinds of discoveries, among them canned condensed milk (which made it possible to give babies milk that was uncontaminated and nutritionally measurable) and rubber (which made possible the invention of the nipple). Breastfeeding, which did not lend itself to scientific or mathematical scrutiny, began to seem old-fashioned and not in keeping with the general science-oriented enlightenment of the times.

Around the turn of the century, primarily for the purpose of going to work or achieving some freedom from the traditional confinement that followed childbirth, women began to use bottles and experiment with prepared formulas. By the 1930s, with growing awareness of the need for bottle steril-ization and improvement of prepared formula, bottle-feeding emerged as a viable and healthy alternative, and, particularly among educated women, literally came into vogue. While some considered bottle-feeding more convenient, what really underscored its popularity was that it was simply more fash-ionable and the mark of higher social status. Studies done in 1955 show that only about 29 percent of newborns were breastfed.

Where does this put us today? Interestingly, since 1970 there has been a revival of breastfeeding, and the parallels with the natural birth movement and new insights into the im-portance of early mother/child contact and the nutritional ad-vantages of breastmilk are not coincidental. The desire for a close bond with their children and the belief that breastmilk provides better nutrition than formula are the reasons most often expressed by women who decide to breastfeed. Provid-ing the baby with immunities against infection, convenience, emotional satisfaction, and the simple fact that it is more nat-ural also feature prominently in the preference for breastfeed-ing. Today over half of newborns are breastfed in the hospital, and 25 percent still receive breastmilk at six months of age.

This is far from a simple turnaround, though. The setting in which women breastfeed today is quite different from that of our predecessors. Our life-styles are not always consistent with traditional full-time mothering, and in this sense we are very much like working women a century ago. The trouble is, we've lost the sources of support and information they had. We don't have a breastfeeding tradition in our immediate past—for the generation of mothers who preceded us, breast-feeding was not the norm. We have to rely more on formal ed-ucation to get the information we need. It's no small task—devising new ways to accommodate both the care of our children and our jobs in a society that is fast-paced, mo-bile, and leaves us geographically separated from our ex-tended families.

Many women discontinue breastfeeding in the early weeks or months of their babies' lives because they either need or want to return to work or school. For them, working and breastfeeding are either too difficult or not permitted. Many who try to continue breastfeeding experience physiological problems caused by separation from their infants, such as decreased milk supply, leakage, and engorgement. Others find little or no support from coworkers and policies at the workplace that sabotage their special needs as breastfeeding mothers. Those who work and breastfeed successfully do so with the encouragement of medical practitioners, family, friends, husbands, and a social and work environment that is positive and supportive.

Most women decide whether or not to breastfeed either before or during their pregnancy. How prepared you are will make a big difference in how smoothly breastfeeding begins and progresses. The American Academy of Pediatrics, which strongly advocates breastfeeding, stresses the importance of getting support and advice from professionals who can offer accurate, up-to-date information. Ultimately, though, the reasons for choosing to breastfeed belong to you—a personal and free choice you make to feed your baby this way.

Your knowledge of the breastfeeding process and its benefits, and your belief that what you are doing is best for your baby, will form the heart of your commitment in the exciting weeks and months ahead. If you are thinking about working and breastfeeding, you'll need to be a bit of an overachiever. The combination of working and parenting is tough enough; add breastfeeding, and you add a host of other challenges, to say the least. But it can be done, and throughout this book you will hear from women who have done it. The experiences and suggestions shared here are meant to give you encouragement and a wealth of invaluable ideas, but they are not meant as absolute prescriptions or as reasons to feel badly if breastfeeding does not work out for you. On the other hand, the more you know, the better your chances are of making the decision—to breastfeed or not—that is right for you.

First of all, in order to design a working/breastfeeding routine that matches both your needs and the baby's needs, a thorough understanding of the physiology and mechanics of breastfeeding is essential.

ADVANTAGES OF BREASTFEEDING

Bonding

Long before there was a word to describe it, women have been reaching out to touch, caress, and gaze at their newborns the instant after birth. Now *bonding* is a part of our everyday birth vocabulary, and in fact, it comes at the top of the list of the reasons women choose to breastfeed. What, exactly, is bonding, and why is it so important?

A short historical excursion is relevant here. Back when most babies were born at home, it was natural to unite mother and infant immediately after birth. The father, too, was likely to be close at hand, along with siblings and other members of the family. During the past several decades, however, in an effort to reduce maternal and infant complications and deaths, birth was moved into the hospital, where a controlled environment and medical expertise are available. A new model for child-birth emerged, one that usually called for isolation of babies from families in the interest of a hospital routine designed to provide optimum sterility. In the late 1960s, research into the effect of parent/infant attachment suggested that separation of babies might be good for excising germs, but not so good for families. The landmark studies of maternal/infant bonding conducted by pediatricians Marshall Klaus and John Kennell showed that mothers who had immediate and extended contact with their babies after birth exhibited stronger attachment and more affectionate behavior toward their infants.

As consumer demand swelled, hospitals began to make changes to get mothers and newborns back together. At the same time, though, misconceptions about bonding caused confusion. Bonding was likened to gluing: If you didn't grab your baby and quickly apply the magic epoxy, your chance for a meaningful relationship with your child was lost. So doctors placed babies on their mothers' skin after birth, fathers were invited to hold and bathe their newborns, and parents were allowed to spend some time in the special "bonding room." And that supposedly did it; the job was thought to be complete.

Bonding as a speedy ritual is far from what Klaus and Kennell, or any of their colleagues, had in mind. Bonding is not an isolated episode, nor is it a fleeting moment in time that we must capture and preserve with Super Glue. It is an ongoing process of loving, caring, and nurturing. True, the emotional excitement of birth, as well as a physiological peak aroused in mothers by postbirth hormones is most intense right after birth. But this is only the beginning of a lifetime of opportunities to touch hearts with our child.

Whether or not you decide to breastfeed, it is both natural and humane for you to hold and be with your infant as soon as possible after birth, and as often as you can in the hours and days that follow. Breastfeeding is an added opportunity for the closest possible physical contact, and your baby craves and needs your skin, your smell, your warmth, your taste, and the loving look she sees in your eyes when you return her gaze. She depends on you—you are the sole source of her nourishment—and you depend on her. Her suckling is what stimulates your body to increase milk production. Each of her feedings will stimulate your body to replenish the supply and ensure that she has enough. Suckling is relaxing and soothing to your baby, and the feeling of relief that comes with easing the pressure of your full breasts will soon be a pleasurable experience for you, too. Your relationship becomes wonderfully reciprocal, and at times perfectly synchronized as you both get better at it.

No wonder we want to keep breastfeeding when we go back to work! When you're separated from your baby for most of the day, breastfeeding gives you optimum intimacy with her when you do reunite. You give continuity to your baby's life, and she learns to rely on you and begins to see the world as a friendly place she can trust. The moment you see her, whether it is midday during your lunch break or when you return home after a full day's work, you will hold her and eagerly connect with her in the closest possible way.

This is not to say that these things won't happen if you don't breastfeed. Breastfeeding has never been shown to be a prerequisite to bonding, the absolute guarantee of a stronger attachment, or the promise of a tantrum-free toddler. What we do know is that breastfeeding provides the ultimate contact with the baby, one that gives pleasure and fulfills emotional and physical needs at the same time. For the women who choose it, breastfeeding is a natural and loving way to nourish their infants—and a choice that deserves a prominent and legitimate time and place in their workdays.

Nutrition

If you are healthy and eating a well-balanced diet, you will produce milk that is nearly a perfect food for your baby. It contains the right amounts of all the vitamins and nutrients for normal growth. (Note: The water-soluble vitamins in human milk are a function of the mother's diet and can be deficient if her diet is deficient.) Breastmilk is the easiest to digest as well as the most efficiently absorbed of any type of infant food. Breastfed babies tend to have loose, non-offensive stools (compared with the firmer, stronger-smelling stools of formula-fed babies), because they are not passing off undigested protein and fat. The amount of iron in breastmilk is lower than that of formula, again because breastfed babies absorb most of what they get. Breastmilk is high in cholesterol, and some researchers theorize that this stimulates the production of enzymes that will in adult life keep cholesterol levels low. Breastmilk contains less sodium and is therefore easier on a newborn's kidneys. The caloric content of your milk comes primarily from lactose (composed of glucose and galactose); lipids (fats); and nitrogen-containing compounds, which appear largely in the form of protein and amino acids.

While there are slight changes in the composition of your milk from day to day (most notably the composition of saturated and polyunsaturated fats, which will be related to your diet), the nutrient base remains fairly constant. The ability of the mother's body to provide just what the baby needs is evidenced by studies of premature infants, which found that the milk of mothers who gave birth prematurely was higher in protein and fat, the very nutrients needed to meet the extra caloric requirement of the low-birthweight babies.

The American Academy of Pediatrics advocates breast-milk as a complete source of nutrition for most babies during the first four to six months of life, with neither supplements nor solid foods necessary during this period. Naturally, there are some exceptions. For example, breastmilk (in fact, all types of milk) is low in vitamin D, and your doctor may recommend a vitamin D supplement, especially during the winter months when the baby is outside less and therefore gets less of this from the sun. Because breastmilk is low in vitamin K, infants born in hospitals receive a vitamin K shot (some out-of-hospital birth centers do not include this procedure). Fluoride is another substance that many doctors suggest be supplemented, whether or not you live in an area with fluoridated water. Vitamin B_{12} deficiencies have been noted in breastfed infants of strict vegetarian (no eggs or dairy products) mothers, but again, no hard and fast rules apply. As for iron, physicians vary in their recommendations of supplements for breastfed babies under six months, though beyond that age, breastfed babies are usually given extra iron through supplements or iron-fortified cereals.

With all the "mays" and "mights," experts generally agree that babies thrive on breastmilk for at least the first six months. Your milk will be ideal for your baby if your diet during pregnancy and lactation is good; you avoid drugs (including alcohol and certain herbal teas and some prescription drugs); you have some caloric reserves tucked away in subcutaneous fat (yes, those extra pounds have a purpose!); and your baby is born with sufficient nutritional stores of her own.

Immunobiology

In the womb, your baby began receiving your immunities through the placenta. These will protect her after birth, while she works on making antibodies of her own. As long as she is nursing, she will receive defenses against diseases to which you have built up an immunity. Even infections you get next week will quickly result in antibodies being transmitted to her via your breastmilk.

For the first three to seven days after birth, your breasts will secrete colostrum, a thick yellowish liquid loaded with antibodies that provide resistance against disease, high in protein and lower in fats and carbohydrates than mature milk. When your milk comes in, it will initially be part milk, part colostrum (called *transitional* milk). In about two weeks your milk will be *mature*, and your baby will digest it easily.

There is impressive evidence to show that breastfed babies have fewer respiratory infections and that babies who are completely breastfed have an intestinal flora, lactobacillus bifidus, that protects them from harmful bacteria. (When solids and/or formula are added to the diet, the flora changes.) Other studies report fewer sick visits to doctors among breastfed babies compared with formula-fed infants. Some researchers have found a lower incidence of SIDS (Sudden Infant Death Syndrome) among breastfed babies, though other studies find no significant correlation.

There are many other elements of human milk that protect babies from both viral and bacterial infections. Still, your breastfed baby may become ill while your neighbor's bottle-fed baby breezes through with nary a sniffle. Remember that your breastfeeding experience may not always conform exactly to scientific theory.

Allergies

There are still many unresolved questions as to whether breastfeeding reduces a child's chances of developing allergies in later life. There is support for the theory that the less exposure an infant has to allergens, the less chance she has of developing seasonal allergies (for example, puffy eyes, sneezing, congestion as a result of dust, pollen, ragweed), asthma, and eczema in later life. Allergy to cow's milk is one of the most common food allergies, and for this reason some physicians do not recommend formulas with a cow's milk base. Even the substitution of soy protein in prepared formulas does not eliminate the risk of allergy, because some babies may be allergic to soy protein.

Breastfeeding is particularly recommended to families who have a history of allergies. This does not necessarily mean you will free your child from all possibility of having adolescent or adult allergies, but you may reduce the odds. If you have an infant who is extremely fussy, or if your family history includes severe allergic reactions, your practitioner might suggest eliminating from your diet possible allergens that could sneak into your breastmilk (eggs, chocolate, cow's milk, and some citrus fruits). However, some of these are very nutritious and should be cut only if the situation absolutely warrants. When the baby is ready for solid foods, some practitioners suggest that you introduce new foods one at a time and at wide intervals, avoiding highly allergenic foods during the first year.

Obesity

It's hard for a breastfed baby to be overfed. When she's full, she quits, and we can't urge her to finish the last few ounces as we might be tempted to do with a bottle. The first milk that comes out of the breast during a feeding is thin and flows freely. As the breast becomes empty, the milk becomes higher in fat. It is possible that this last, richer milk is nature's method of appetite control—the baby feels sated and either stops nursing or sucks less heartily. At this point you usually switch the baby to the other breast, and again she sucks more vigorously at the beginning and slows down near the end. If she does continue sucking at the breast after it is essentially empty, it's mostly for the fun and comfort of it, because the amount of milk she is getting is negligible.

On the issue of the relationship between infant feeding and adult weight problems, much is theorized but little is really known. Some studies show that more obese adults were formula-fed; others show no difference. The introduction of solid foods and inducing a baby to finish a bottle may play bigger roles in causing overweight babies than the formula itself.

Whether or not we predispose babies to adult obesity by fattening them up as infants, thus creating a larger number of fat cells, is not known for sure. It is more likely that the first several years of life are all critical to fat-cell development, and the American Academy of Pediatrics says that excessive weight gain should be avoided not only in infancy but throughout childhood. There are obese breastfed babies, but most practitioners would agree that they should still be fed on demand, and that the fat will disappear later.

Convenience

Breastfeeding is more convenient than bottle-feeding. Your baby is a light traveler—grab a couple of diapers and she can go anywhere with you. Her food supply and source of comfort are only a couple of blouse buttons away. You have no formula to prepare, no bottles to sterilize, no problem finding the right nipple with the right-sized hole, no need to find a place to warm the bottle, no testing to make sure it's the correct temperature.

However, in the first few weeks of your baby's life you might find yourself wondering, Hey, when is this going to get convenient? Breastfed newborns seem to nurse constantly; they take this on-demand schedule seriously. As you roll out of bed in the middle of the night for the second time, knowing your bottle-feeding neighbor is sleeping peacefully, breast-feeding simply doesn't feel easier. But have patience. It may take a couple of weeks for your baby to establish anything that remotely resembles a schedule, but that's exactly what nature has in mind. You and your baby are in the process of synchro-nizing your rhythms. Her frequent feedings are signaling your body to produce more milk so you can keep up with her fast growing needs. In a very short time your baby will go longer between feedings, and your body will be in perfect tune with her hunger. Then, frankly, you won't believe how easy it is!

Now what happens when you go back to work? Sud-denly breastfeeding isn't quite so simple. You are adding com-plications to your day that you would not have if you left your baby with a caregiver and a day's supply of formula. Breast-feeding and working does *not* make your workday easier. The rewards come after work, when you can greet her with a ready source of food and comfort the moment you arrive; at night, when you barely have to open your eyes to pick her up and nurse; and all the other times in between, when every feeding is a chance to relax and take full advantage of the time you have together, with nothing to do but simply enjoy being as close to your baby as you can get.

Getting Back in Shape

An important effect of breastfeeding can be felt almost immediately after birth. The release of oxytocin, caused by your baby's first suckling, triggers contractions of the muscle cells in the uterus, which helps it to return to its prepregnancy size and shape (and with it, your abdomen). This may also re-duce the amount of postpartum bleeding.

It may take as many as five hundred extra calories a day to produce breastmilk. In a sense, breastfeeding is a natural diet. As long as you continue to eat well-balanced foods, you probably won't have to do anything else to lose the extra pounds you picked up during pregnancy. Remember, though, that while you are nursing you should not attempt any kind of crash dieting. Let nature take care of it for you.

When Not to Breastfeed

While there are few contraindications to breastfeeding, they should be mentioned. First of all, any kind of debilitating disease that leaves a mother too ill to breastfeed would be one reason to choose a bottle-feeding alternative. Mothers with active infections such as sputum-positive tuberculosis and hepatitis B virus are restricted from nursing. With careful attention to hand washing and hygiene, mothers with herpes simplex may be allowed to breastfeed. In the rare case of breastmilk jaundice, breastfeeding may be interrupted briefly while the infant is fully examined and the level of serum bilirubin in her blood is evaluated. (This condition is not to be confused with physiological jaundice—which sometimes occurs in the days following birth—when breastfeeding can and should continue.)

You should use extreme caution in taking any medication during lactation, because most drugs are excreted in your milk. Daily aspirin should be used with caution, and only after you have consulted your physician. If you need to take a drug for a specific disease, make sure it is not one known to have adverse effects on your baby, and watch the baby for evidence of side effects. You may need to explore alternative therapy, or at the very least, you should be fully informed about the effects any medication prescribed for you may have on your baby.

While little is known conclusively about the effects of such substances as nicotine, marijuana, and alcohol, these drugs should be avoided. Any drug that alters a mother's state of consciousness could interfere with her ability to care for her baby and should be shunned for this reason alone. Remember that currently there is very little absolute scientific knowledge on the effects of drugs on your baby.

HIV, the virus that causes AIDS, can be transmitted from an infected woman to her fetus or newborn during pregnancy, labor, and delivery, and through breastfeeding, according to the U.S. Public Health Service in its Recommendations for HIV Counseling and Testing for Pregnant Women, February 23, 1995. The statement also estimates that breastfeeding may increase the rate of transmission by 10 to 20 percent. If you are HIV positive, you may want to discuss the bottle-feeding alternative with your doctor.

WOMEN AT WORK

Whatever your reasons for working—from sheer economic necessity to the development of a career—you have a right to do so. Men work while being fathers, and few are ever asked how they "balance family and career."

On the other hand, for most of us there is no question that our children take priority over our jobs. If we feel forced to make choices between job and baby, and the job sometimes wins out, it is because we are stuck in a system that does not accommodate our needs as both mothers and workers. There is simply no excuse in this country and this era for the discrimination that occurs in the workplace against parents. As a nation, we cry out how much we care about children. But in the day-to-day lives of most parents, we are consistently asked to put our children's needs aside for the good of the company, the business, the economy.

Throughout the world, the voices of women who wish to combine working and breastfeeding are gradually being heard. A number of industrialized nations have programs and policies specifically set up to harmonize working and breastfeeding, such as extended maternity or parental leaves with pay. In Uruguay, mothers can work half-time in order to breastfeed during their babies' first six months. Mothers receive full salary. At some worksites in Mozambique, India, and Thailand, crèches are provided near the workplace so that mothers can breastfeed. In the Philippines, one child care service provides wetnursing. Breastfeeding mothers there manage the center and breastfeed their own babies as well as other babies.

The Innocenti Declaration on the Protection, Promotion, and Support of Breastfeeding was adopted by participants at the WHO/UNICEF meeting on breastfeeding held at the Spedale degli Innocenti, Florence, Italy, in August of 1990. The declaration, signed by thirty governments, states that all women should be enabled to breastfeed exclusively, and infants should be fed breastmilk exclusively from birth to four to six months. The declaration calls on nations to enact legislation protecting the rights of working/breastfeeding women, and to curtail the marketing of breastmilk substitutes to working women. At the recent United Nations Conference on Women, delegates noted that "restrictive work arrangements, social stigma, and false information are denying [women] a choice in how to feed their babies."

In an article entitled "When Private Goes Public: Legal Protection for Women Who Breastfeed in Public and at Work" (*Law and Inequality: A Journal of Theory and Practice,* December, 1995), author Danielle M. Shelton writes: "Breastfeeding women wonder whether they will be harassed, evicted, or even arrested for feeding their babies in public. Moreover, employed breastfeeding women worry about whether and how they can breastfeed or breastpump at work." Shelton cites U.S. Bureau of Labor statistics showing that over 50 percent of mothers with children under the age of three are working outside the home. Among mothers who work full-time, more than half begin breastfeeding in the hospital, yet only 12.5 percent are still nursing five to six months later, in contrast to nearly 23 percent of mothers nursing who are at home. Shelton writes: "When breastfeeding women leave their homes and attempt to integrate breastfeeding into their public and professional lives, they face barriers to breastfeeding that require legal protection."

The most we have been able to accomplish so far in the U.S. is the Family and Medical Leave Act, a federal law passed in 1993. This law gives those who work for companies with fifty or more employees the right to take up to twelve weeks of unpaid leave a year to care for a newborn or newly adopted child, a seriously ill family member, or to recover from a serious health condition, including pregnancy.

State initiatives to assist breastfeeding mothers have been slow, but there are some. Twelve states have either passed or are considering legislation concerning breastfeeding mothers, according to a 1995 article entitled "Out of the Mouths of Babies: No Mother's Milk for U.S. Children," by Isabelle Schallreuter Olson in the Winter 1995 issue of *Hamline Law Review.* These laws vary in content and scope from protecting a breastfeeding woman for indecent exposure to excluding her from jury duty. New York is the only state to classify breastfeeding as a civil right. More about state laws to promote breastfeeding, the Family and Medical Leave Act, and legal protection for breastfeeding mothers follows in Chapter Eleven.

We're a long way from an ideal system. First, it is necessary for our culture to promote and support breastfeeding as a truly viable choice. Then, we must be willing to commit funds, employ staff, and enact policies and legislation toward providing an environment that is friendly to that choice—one that simplifies the logistics of breastfeeding and working by offering flexible scheduling, extended parental leaves and benefits, child care, on-site nursing care for infants, and an official imprimatur of advocacy and encouragement. Until then, the movement toward working and breastfeeding will be the spontaneous, individual effort of persons like you—women willing to maneuver through the system, or in some cases sidetrack it—and in doing so, begin to tread a path for those grateful parents who follow.

2

Breastfeeding Basics

"The body is an incredible thing. It seems to be able to fix just about any problem that comes up in breastfeeding. When the baby needs more, you produce more; when the baby needs less, you produce less. The body does it. I wish I could have relaxed more—it would have been easier."

When you become pregnant, your breasts are usually the first to know. From the moment of conception, they start getting ready to provide your baby's food. In fact, one of the earliest signs that you were pregnant was probably the enlargement, tenderness, tingling, and darkening of the areola (the area around the nipple). Actually, your breasts have been gearing up for milk production since adolescence, when they began to grow and take shape. While you were worrying about filling out your bathing suit, your breasts were busy developing the apparatus of lactation, and by the time you were in your mid-teens (earlier for some young women), they were ready to support another life.

Milk production begins deep in the breast, where clusters of cells called alveoli take ingredients from the bloodstream and turn them into milk. The alveoli are connected to a richly branched system of milk ducts. These ducts come together into reservoirs called lactiferous sinuses, where milk is stored. When the baby suckles, the milk travels from the reservoirs through another set of ducts and then gently sprays out through many tiny openings in the nipple. While the number of openings varies from woman to woman (from fifteen to twenty-five if you're counting), neither this nor the size of your breasts affects your ability to produce or give milk. Small breasts do just as well as large ones.

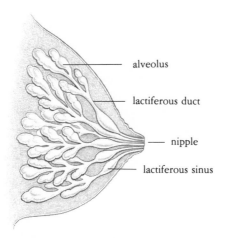

alveolus

lactiferous duct

nipple

lactiferous sinus

Nipples also vary. But in spite of what your mother may have told you about some women not being able to nurse because their nipples were "wrong," there are actually very few instances where a nipple problem prevents a woman from nursing. Some women have what are called inverted nipples, but with a little extra attention (discussed later in the chapter) this can be corrected in most cases.

How Milk Is Produced

The main player in milk production is a hormone called prolactin, which is produced by the pituitary gland, located in your brain. Your body produces small amounts of prolactin all the time, but when you are pregnant the amount increases considerably. The reason you don't make milk during pregnancy is that two other hormones, estrogen and progesterone, keep the levels of prolactin in check. At the time of birth, the levels of estrogen and progesterone drop dramatically, allowing prolactin to swing into action and begin stimulating the milk supply.

When your baby is nursing, nerves in the nipple send impulses to the pituitary gland telling it to release more prolactin. This in turn stimulates the milk-producing cells to make milk. Since the breast does not keep huge reserves of milk, this constant emptying of the breast and restimulation of the prolactin supply is necessary to keep the whole process going. This is also the way the baby lets your body know how much milk is needed, and the way your body keeps up with your baby's growing demands. In the early days of your baby's life, frequent nursing will build up your milk supply. As time goes by, your baby will nurse less often, but regular intervals are necessary to maintain the balance between what your baby needs and what you produce.

As a working/nursing mother, maintaining this balance between supply and demand will be the most important part of your daily strategy. If it is necessary for you to miss feedings and you want to maintain a total milk supply for the baby, you will need to manually express the milk your baby would ordinarily have taken at those feedings. Otherwise, your body won't get enough milk-producing messages and your baby's needs will outdistance your supply. However, it is also possible to adjust production to skip feedings (providing formula in your absence), and many women choose this method. Because later chapters focus specifically on timing and the techniques used in expressing breastmilk and managing your daily schedule, for now we will stay with what happens in the early weeks as the supply and demand become synchronized.

Colostrum and First Milk

Around the fourth month of your pregnancy your breasts began making colostrum, a thick yellowish substance that you may have noticed occasionally leaking from your breasts sometime in the second trimester. Colostrum is the first food your baby will receive and, as discussed in Chapter One, it is loaded with antibodies and nutrients to give your baby extra protection and a special boost to start life outside the womb. Colostrum is lower than milk in fats and higher in protein. The laxative effect of colostrum helps clear the intestinal tract of meconium (those undelightful sticky black first stools). Your baby gets mere teaspoons of colostrum—much less than the milk that will come in later. Not getting full causes the baby to nurse more often, which helps stimulate the milk supply, and also ensures that she gets plenty of colostrum.

About three to seven days after birth, your milk will "come in." Your breasts may swell and feel tender and full. When you first begin producing milk, the swelling is due largely to increased blood and fluids in the breast tissue. If they become hard and painful to the touch, this is called, appropriately, engorgement. Engorgement, which is common but not inevitable, can sometimes be avoided by increased feedings.

When her milk first came in, recalls Donna R., "It wasn't as painful as people said it was going to be, but it was pretty painful. My breasts got really hard, and I noticed that in the mirror the veins in them were really prominent. They felt huge and full. And my breasts felt really hot. When it was time to nurse her again, I knew the milk had come in because when I'd take her away to burp her I'd see milk instead of colostrum."

"When my milk came in at the hospital I was just ecstatic," Melissa B. says. "I couldn't believe it. I was pretty flat before—an A inverted. Afterward, it was a *B*—for me, that was a big deal."

Nursing soon after birth and as frequently as possible (every two to three hours or more in the daytime and every four to five hours at night) will help shorten this engorgement phase of lactation. Sometimes the swelling causes the nipple to become flat and difficult for the baby to grasp. Hand or pump expression of some milk before the feeding will soften the breast and make the nipple more accessible. A warm bath or shower, or a warm cloth on the breasts, will also help to start the milk flowing. It is a good idea to nurse on both breasts at each feeding, allowing about five to ten minutes per side, with a burp in between. But use these times as general guidelines only. Your baby may want to linger at the breast, and you may want to turn your wristwatch facedown and follow her signals instead. Later, if you develop sore or cracked nipples, you may need to reduce the nursing time, but we will cross that bridge later in the chapter when we discuss specific problems.

The first real milk you produce (the transitional milk) is thick and rich and light yellow in color, though still mixed with colostrum. Within ten days to two weeks, your milk will change again, becoming thin and watery and white, gray, or light blue in color. This mature milk may have you wondering, since it doesn't look at all like the bottled stuff we buy in the store. But as with each phase of your milk supply, this product is perfectly suited to your baby's needs, and its lighter composition (due to a higher water content) is one of the reasons it is easier on your baby's kidneys and liver than formula or cow's milk.

The Let-Down Reflex

Let's go back to what happens when your baby suckles. Among the messages sent from the nerves in the nipple to the pituitary gland is one that stimulates the release of oxytocin, a hormone that causes the muscles around the milk cells to contract and eject the milk into the reservoirs, out the nipple, and into your baby's mouth. When the milk lets down well, the baby is more likely to get both the thinner *fore milk* (first to come out) and the richer, high calorie *hind milk*. If you have never nursed before, it might take a minute or two for the let-down reflex to work. As your baby suckles, you may feel the milk rush in with a pleasant, tingling sensation. On the other hand, you might not feel anything at all. This is also normal and does not mean your let-down reflex isn't working. A good indication that the reflex is working is the sound of your baby gulping or a spurt or leakage of milk from the non-nursing breast. "It's a kind of burning sensation—little tingling pins—like when your arm goes to sleep and is trying to wake up," says Katie, a first-time mother. "If I'm exercising or out shopping and she's home with her dad, I can tell when it's time to get home!"

As time goes by, your let-down reflex will become quite efficient, and the milk flow will begin almost as soon as your baby's mouth hits the nipple—or before. Some women let down when they hear their babies cry; others do so while turning into the driveway after work. On occasion you may be so attuned to your baby that a passing thought about that sweet little cherub miles away brings milk gushing in. This can be disconcerting, particularly if you leak all over your blouse in the middle of a business luncheon. But if you are away from your baby at a regular feeding time, your breasts, creatures of habit that they are, simply go ahead on their own. It helps to establish a regular routine of hand or pump expression during the workday, and you may want to keep breast pads handy to absorb leakage. As the supply/demand rhythm becomes more predictable, you will experience fewer incidences of un-scheduled let-down; you will also learn how often you need to express to make sure you produce the right amount of milk at the right times. And as mentioned earlier, some working women are able to adjust their supply to a routine that does not necessitate expression: They nurse while at home and provide formula while at work.

A free-spirited, strong let-down reflex is not universal. Some mothers experience let-down problems, particularly at first. Embarrassment, stress, physical pain, and anxiety about nursing can interfere with the flow of milk, and these problems can occur periodically even with the most seasoned breastfeeders.

If your let-down reflex is not working, try to relax. Oh sure, you say, but how? First of all, make sure you're physically comfortable. Put your feet up, and play some relaxing music. Sit in a rocker. Prop a pillow under your arm or in your lap. Seek some privacy, if you need it. Have a drink of something you like (avoid too many caffeine drinks, such as coffee or soda). Take some deep breaths—the kind you learned in childbirth class. A warm bath or shower before the feeding may help, as will warm wet compresses on the breast or a hand massage of the nipples. Sometimes running warm water over your hands or stroking a soft object will stimulate the let-down. Look at your baby and caress her beautiful brand-new skin or her little downy head. When you put your baby to the breast, the nipple should be completely in her mouth so that her lips are pressed against the areola and her chin is right against the breast. Gently pinch the areola with your fingertips to make it easier for the baby to grasp.

One more word about oxytocin. You'll be happy to know that this hormone also stimulates the uterus to contract to its original prepregnancy size and shape. You may feel mild or even severe cramps (called afterpains) the first few times you breastfeed, a signal that you have an active let-down reflex and that a flat stomach is just around the corner. Afterpains become more intense with successive births. Sometimes normal post-birth bleeding increases during nursing, again because the uterus is contracting. Occasionally, a severely stubborn let-down reflex can be stimulated by the use of a nasal spray containing oxytocin, though this requires a prescription and has been known to cause headaches in some women who have used it.

Is There Enough Milk?

If we had transparent breasts, we could measure the milk and know the baby was getting enough. As it is, we must trust in the process. But it is an efficient process, indeed, a simple balance of supply and demand. The more you nurse, the more milk you will make. Every time your baby suckles, the nerves in the nipple send a signal to the brain to step up production of milk. As long as you nurse frequently and eat enough good foods, your body will maintain a supply that matches your baby's needs.

The best way to make sure you have an ample supply of milk is to nurse on demand, that is, whenever your baby wants to. Some babies nurse every hour at first, and during the early weeks, expect your baby to nurse every hour and a half to two hours during the day (although most babies quickly fall into a fairly predictable schedule, with longer intervals between feedings and fewer feedings at night). Remember, your baby's frequent nursing is the way your milk supply is built up. If you supplement with formula, your breasts will not make enough, and your supply could lag behind your baby's appetite. This can become a vicious circle; the more you supplement, the less milk you produce and the more you need to supplement. Bottles, especially during the early weeks, are one of the main culprits in disruption of the supply/demand balance.

Nursing right after birth stimulates the lactation hormones, as well as the release of oxytocin to help the uterus contract. But besides getting breastfeeding off to the best possible start, this immediate contact with your baby is what you both want and need. The research on bonding conducted by Klaus and Kennell (discussed in Chapter One) showed that babies who nursed during the first hour after birth continued breastfeeding longer that those who did not have this early opportunity.

If you are giving birth in a hospital, advise your practitioner in advance that you wish to nurse on the delivery table. Make sure the hospital's policies are flexible, supportive, and do not separate you from your baby unnecessarily. It is now considered medically acceptable to delay for up to two hours the administration of 1 percent silver nitrate to the newborn's eyes. Since these drops impair vision and interfere with the infant's first eye contact, you can request this short postponement. Some states permit tetracycline or erythromycin as alternatives to silver nitrate. These, too, can be postponed for two hours since they also impair the baby's vision.

Rooming-in will enable you to nurse and cuddle your baby as often as you like, but if this is not an option, make sure the hospital routine encourages nursing on demand, frequently, and throughout the night. Your baby does not need to be given water or formula in the nursery. If supplementing is for some reason medically necessary, it should be carried out by written request only. Some hospitals bring breastfed babies to the mother with a bottle in the carrier. Don't be intimidated by this implication that you may not have enough milk. A lot of suckling at the breast is essential to the development of a good milk supply. Supplements in the early days can subvert the initiation of a good supply/demand balance.

As we mentioned before, your newborn will want to nurse quite often. Sometimes you'll wonder why you even bother to rebutton your blouse. Pretty soon you'll be thinking: "Demand" is certainly the word for it! And if you just nursed an hour ago, can there be any milk there at all? When your baby is on a short interval, your breasts may not feel full, but there is enough milk inside. And because you are breastfeeding frequently, your body is making plenty more.

During these tiring times it helps to remember that this is exactly what is supposed to happen—your baby and your body are in the process of becoming beautifully and perfectly synchronized. Before long the intervals will increase, and breastfeeding will be a breeze. In the meantime, relax and realize that feeding your baby is the biggest part of your job as a new parent. Forget about the household needs, your job, entertaining friends, and treat yourself to activities that put you in a peaceful, relaxed state of mind—reading, listening to music, talking with friends on the phone, watching television. Rely on your partner for household chores. Your baby needs to be close to you, to study your face, feel your heartbeat, to snuggle safely in your big warm arms. What else is there for you to do that can be more important than that?

Like adults, babies have days when they are hungrier than others. They also have several growth spurts, usually at about two weeks, at four to six weeks, and again at around three months. During these times, your baby will want to nurse very often, almost constantly it seems, for a period lasting about forty-eight hours. Hang in there! Your baby is growing and needs more food, and this sudden run on your milk is nature's way of beefing up your supply in anticipation of an older, bigger baby. After a day or so, you will settle down to a regular routine again. Studies have shown that it takes about two days of ample suckling to increase the milk supply.

As a working/nursing mother, you will need to be particularly concerned with supply and demand. If your milk production is in harmony with your baby's needs before you return to work, you will have less difficulty keeping pace with your baby even though you will be away for some feedings. By the time you return to work, the interval between feedings will be longer, and you will have a good idea how much milk you need to express manually in order to maintain production.

You Can Tell If Your Baby Is Getting Enough Milk . . .

- If she has one wet diaper for each day of life in the first week.
- If she has six or more wet cloth diapers a day (and is not getting any extra water).
- If she is nursing eight to ten times every twenty-four hours (at least once during the night).

- If she has three to four heavy diapers a day after the first week.
- If she is at birth weight at two weeks (Babies normally lose weight the first week and then regain it).
- If she is gaining weight—about a pound or more a month after the second week. (Note: breastfed babies usually gain at a slower rate than bottle-fed babies.)
- If she has a healthy skin color and tone.

GETTING STARTED

Preparation for breastfeeding begins during pregnancy. The best source of information and support is other mothers who have breastfed, particularly those who have continued to breastfeed after returning to work. If you have never watched a woman breastfeed a baby, find one and spend some time with her. If you don't have any friends or friends-of-friends currently breastfeeding, ask your childbirth instructor or birth practitioner for the names of newly delivered mothers who might be willing to let you drop by during a feeding. Most mothers are happy to share their experiences and help smooth the way for someone else.

It is essential to have the support of your partner. If you don't, this does not mean you shouldn't breastfeed, but you will have to be extra committed to compensate for his lack of enthusiasm. Encourage him to talk about his concerns, and share in the reading of books and information you find helpful. Suggest that he talk with other "breastfeeding fathers." The more enthusiastic and committed you are, the more likely it is that your attitude will rub off on him.

Is your birth practitioner an advocate of breastfeeding? Look around the office on your first visit. Is a wide selection of breastfeeding literature prominently displayed? Does the bulletin board have notices of prepared childbirth classes and La Leche League schedules (an international organization that offers information and support to breastfeeding mothers)? Plan to discuss your wish for immediate breastfeeding and frequent contact with your baby during your hospital stay. Is an out-of-hospital birthing center an option for you? If your inquiries do not elicit a positive, supportive response, you may want to change practitioners, or at least be sure you feel assertive enough to insist on the kind of birth experience you want.

It is equally important to select a pediatrician early, and to find one who is supportive and informed about breastfeeding. Schedule a prenatal interview and ask lots of questions. Many mothers-to-be visit several pediatricians before selecting one, and these prenatal visits are customarily offered at no charge. At this stage, you can also learn quite a bit about a pediatrician by talking with mothers of other patients. If you learn that he is quick to advise supplements any time a mother hits a snag, or that he routinely prescribes solid foods to breastfed babies early (before four to six months), you may be dealing with a doctor who is not wholeheartedly in favor of breastfeeding. Either change doctors or simply be aware that you may not always follow his advice. Many parents don't have trouble with this; others have difficulty challenging a pediatrician where their newborn is concerned. If you are in the latter category, you might be better off choosing another practitioner. Find one who believes, as does the American Academy of Pediatrics, that breastmilk is the only food a baby needs for the first four to six months and that a baby can be breastfed for a year.

Prenatal Nutrition and Weight Gain

During your pregnancy, you will want to follow all the guidelines of good prenatal nutrition advised by your birth practitioner. Generally, a weight gain of at least twenty-five pounds is desirable, though some women gain more. Remember that much of the extra fat you put on during pregnancy is in storage specifically for the purpose of lactation. It will seem to melt away as you continue to nurse, and you may find that you can eat everything you need and still lose the pounds you gained during pregnancy. It may take about five hundred additional calories a day to make milk, so as long as you don't take up the slack in Snickers bars, breastfeeding may be the best diet you ever tried. Be patient—it often takes from three to six months to get back to your prepregnancy weight. Some women don't lose all the weight until after they finish nursing, others never lose it all.

Bras

During your fifth or sixth month of pregnancy (earlier if you have already outgrown your regular bras), you will need to shop for larger, well-fitting bras to accommodate and support your increasing breast size. Taking care of your breasts in this way will reduce the chances of stretch marks (though many women get them anyway because of the rapid growth) and sagging later on. Many women begin wearing nursing bras at this time; others prefer to stick with prenatal bras until shortly before term, when they have a better idea of the size their nursing breasts will be. Prenatal bras are very much like regular bras but provide much more support, which is essential during this period. It is a good idea to buy two, because if you try to get by on one, it's likely to get laundered to death and lose its valuable support more quickly. If your girth increases but the cup size stays the same, you can add a bra extender, which hooks to the bra fasteners to lengthen the girth. You may be able to use your prenatal bras later, after you stop nursing.

Nursing bras cost a few dollars more than prenatal bras. If you do decide to go right into nursing bras at five months, you might still have to buy a larger size at the end of your pregnancy. While some women stay the same size throughout, most experience an increase in size, especially when the milk comes in. If you wait until you are midway between your eighth and ninth month to buy nursing bras, and have them carefully fitted by an experienced retailer or salesperson, they will last through the first few months of nursing. The girth should be fitted to allow for reduction after birth.

Both prenatal and nursing bras are designed to grow one

size with you, provided they are fitted properly to begin with. The number size of the bra does not always correspond to the size you wore before you became pregnant, and sizes also vary among styles. Don't wait until the baby is born and send your spouse to the store with the mission of bringing back a 34 C. Your chances of getting a good fit are slim.

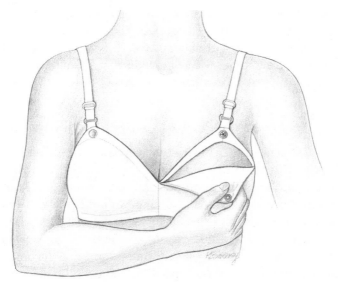

One type of nursing bra

As you shop in the maternity departments of large stores or in small maternity shops, you'll find a number of bra styles. Some have a flap that lets down; others open at the center. Your decision here will be a matter of personal preference, but try to find one with an enclosure clip that you can undo with one hand. Then you won't have to lay the baby down while you fumble with the flap to get to the food.

The bra should give plenty of support, with neither gaps nor places where it cuts into the breast. It should be comfortably snug at the bottom and sufficiently loose-fitting not to be uncomfortable when your pregnancy advances and the umbilicus rises. It should not be so tight that it flattens the nipples. About a pinch of extra fabric in the cup will allow enough room for additional growth or for expansion when your milk comes in. If it is any slacker than that, the support is diminished. As for fabric, this, too, is a matter of preference. Some women are sensitive to lace and nylon, and prefer 100 percent cotton or a cotton blend. Because plastic liners trap moisture and restrict the air to the nipple, they should not be worn in the cup routinely but can be worn for short periods, for example, if you want to protect good clothing. A safety pin can come in handy—attach it to your bra to remind you which side to begin with on the next feeding. You can also use masking tape to do the job.

Nipple Preparation

If you have an ordinary protracted nipple (one that sticks out), you don't have to do anything special to get ready to nurse. Nipple preparation may not help to toughen the nipples, but it will get you accustomed to handling your breasts. This is particularly important for working mothers who want to do a lot of manual expression of milk. While supporting the breast with one hand, use the thumb and first finger of the other hand to gently pull the nipple and roll it between the thumb and finger. Then rotate the position on the nipple and repeat. Repeat this exercise five or six times, several times each day while dressing, at bedtime, or in the bath. Caution: Avoid stroking too long or too hard, as this may stimulate premature contractions.

Some nipples are flat, or inverted. They are difficult for a baby to grasp. In spite of any old wives' tales you may have heard, these nipples are perfectly capable of breastfeeding but, like a shy person, they simply need to be drawn out a little. If it doesn't stick out, you may have a flat nipple. Inverted nipples shrink inward.

The Hoffman technique can be used by all women but is especially designed to draw out flat or inverted nipples. Place either your thumbs or your index fingers opposite each other on the sides of the nipple. Gently draw them away from each other, stretching the areola. Then place the thumbs or fingers above and below the nipple and repeat the stretching maneuver. Do this at least once a day, twice during the last six weeks of pregnancy.

Breast shields can be worn inside the bra during pregnancy and after birth to draw out the nipples. Breast shields, also called breast shells, breast cups, or Woolwich shields, are made of hard, lightweight plastic. They have two parts. An inner ring puts pressure on the areola to draw out the nipple, and the second, domed part holds the bra away from the nipple. Breast shields can also be used to protect sore, cracked nipples, but either use the ones with air holes, or make sure you give the nipples plenty of time to dry after a feeding. Also, use of breast shields can contribute to engorgement, by compressing the breast. If you leak milk into a breast shield, discard the milk and wash the shield.

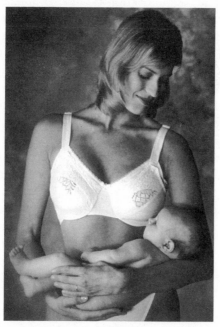

Medela Nursing Bra

Rubber breast shields can be worn during nursing, however, and in this case combine with the baby's suckling to protract the nipples. You can also add a rubber nipple to the plastic shield. But because direct mouth-to-nipple contact is important to trigger the release of lactation hormones, it is best to limit the use of the breast shield to the first part of the nursing, then remove the shield and place the baby directly on the nipple.

Nipples do not usually need creams during pregnancy or after birth. The breasts lubricate themselves naturally through the Montgomery glands, the tiny pimple-like bumps on the areola. However, if the nipples do become dry or cracked, small amounts of lanolin or vitamin E can be used to soothe the nipple and areola (do not use lotions that contain alcohol or an antiseptic, and do not use lanolin if you are allergic to wool). Avoid using soap on the nipples, as this can dry them out, and don't rub them vigorously with a towel. Pat them dry instead. Fresh air, sunlight (not too much), and sexual foreplay with the breasts are all excellent preparations for nursing.

Many experts believe that modern women tend to get cracked and sore nipples because they wear bras all of the time. The bra protects the nipple from the normal friction of rubbing against looser clothing. You might keep this in mind, and make sure you give your breasts lots of fresh air, sunshine, and free time out of the bra.

What are your chances of getting cracked nipples? It's an old wives' tale that if you are fair skinned or red-headed, you stand a greater chance of being sore at first. But most women, particularly those who don't time the feedings with a stopwatch but let the baby nurse as long as she wants, report soreness or pain at some time or another during the early days or weeks of lactation. And almost all of these mothers say it was a temporary discomfort "that would have happened sooner or later anyway—why not get it over with?" We'll discuss how to care for sore nipples in the section on "Common Problems" (page 41).

While nipple preparation may reduce the severity of soreness or cracking, the best way to avoid problems is to position the baby correctly (see following section, "The First Feeding").

The First Feeding

Everywhere in the world, and for all the centuries of birth, infants have been going to the breast immediately after birth. Your baby can be placed at the breast as soon as her airway has been gently suctioned to remove the mucus and she is breathing well on her own. (By the way, newborn infants breathe very erratically—after all, this is their first try at it.) The cord may or may not be clamped and cut first.

Skin-to-skin contact is important for your baby and for you, but if the room is chilly, a loose cover can be placed over the baby for warmth. You'll need some extra hands to help you get settled comfortably and to support the baby beside you. Most women prefer to lie on their side for the first nursing. With your free hand, cup your breast and gently grasp the area behind the nipple to make it protrude. Stroke the baby's lower lip with the nipple. This will stimulate the baby's rooting reflex, and she will turn her head toward the stroke in search of the nipple. (Isn't instinct beautiful?) Insert the nipple into her mouth, getting as much of it and the areola in as possible without stuffing. In the correct position, the lips clamp the areola and the tongue thrusts forward and moves rhythmically in and out to draw the nipple and areola into the mouth. The breast is milked by the forward position of the tongue and its up and down motion as it compresses the nipple against the hard palate.

This may sound unnecessarily mechanistic, but it is important to understand suckling so you can recognize if your baby is not suckling properly. If she suckles only the nipple, it is both painful for you and inefficient for her. Unless the breast is correctly milked, your baby won't get enough, and your production will not be stimulated. If your baby does not get enough of the areola into her mouth the first time, or if her tongue is not forward, break the suction by placing your finger in the corner of her mouth (don't pull her off the breast—ouch!) and try again.

Margot L. remembers: "Nobody really instructed me; the nurses just assumed I knew how to do it. Then after I got home, Brian kept crying a lot, and I just thought the milk hadn't come in. But my breasts were getting real tender, and when he nursed it really hurt a lot. I got to where I was even using breathing techniques because it hurt so bad. I just assumed my nipples weren't ready for it, that they were just tender. Finally my mom said something was wrong, so we headed into town to try to find an answer. First we went to the hospital, because the doctor's office was closed that day. The hospital suggested one of those nipple shields, so we went to the drugstore to get that and to get some special lotion. The whole time we had a book we were reading to try to find an answer there, and I read that you have to push the full nipple and areola into his mouth. I was just putting the tip in. So when we got home with all the other things, I sat down to nurse him and put the whole area [areola] of the nipple in, and it was great! He just drank and drank and drank, and went to sleep and slept so soundly. And I didn't suffer any soreness of my nipples or anything. Such a simple thing, but if you didn't know it, real difficult."

If you are engorged at first, this can flatten the areola and make the nipple hard to grasp. Manual expression of some milk will soften the areola and allow the nipple to protract. And although your baby's chin should be pressed snugly against your breast, her nose should not. You may need to use your finger to press the breast away from the nasal opening; if she can't breathe, she sure can't nurse, and she'll let you know by squirming and acting very frustrated.

Don't be upset if your baby doesn't plunge in immediately. During the first few nursings, expression of a drop of colostrum on the baby's lips can sometimes awaken her interest and get her started. Some babies are eager and efficient from the start, while others dally around and show only mild interest until the milk comes in. Some like to taste and sample the nipple before they latch on; others stop now and then for a break or a short snooze. It's important to follow your baby's pace. Don't rush or prod her. If she falls asleep at the first breast, you may want to wake her after a while (change her diaper or play with her) and switch her to the other breast.

How long should you nurse at first? Opinions vary, but five minutes at each side seems to be a popular figure, with gradual increases. However, your baby may want to linger for as long as twenty minutes or more. It's up to you. If your nipples become sore, you may have to shorten the nursing time until the problem clears up. Don't worry too much about the clock, and don't try to anticipate scheduling. Your baby's routine will change daily during the first few weeks, and the more you can go with the flow (pun intended), the more attuned you and your baby will become. Eventually your newborn will settle into a fairly predictable schedule—in plenty of time for you to plan your return to work. For now, relax and feed your baby as often as you wish. If you don't have rooming-in, you will want to make arrangements in advance to have your baby brought to you at frequent intervals, preferably whenever she is hungry.

Some hospitals will take the liberty of giving the baby water in the middle of the night so you can sleep. However, this causes you to miss valuable milk-stimulation time, and the use of a rubber nipple can confuse the baby and interfere with her development of a good suckling reflex at the breast. Ask to be awakened.

Nurse from both breasts at each feeding, alternating the breast you begin with. The baby may not be very interested at first, but she should be offered the breast every one and one-half to two hours. Since you may be slightly full, you'll welcome these emptyings, and of course, each nursing ensures that your supply will keep up with the demand (see "Engorgement," page 40).

If you give birth in a birthing center, you may be able to come home within a few hours and begin settling in right away. If you spend several days in the hospital, when you come home you may experience some upheaval in whatever rhythm you may have established during your stay. First of all, the excitement and flurry of the discharge and the arrival home can upset both you and your baby. Try to make the transition as smooth as possible. The first day home, your baby may want to nurse quite often. Relax, drink to thirst, welcome the attentions of anyone who wants to pamper you, and lie back and nurse your baby. During the next few weeks, you'll be surprised how quickly your baby will begin to show signs of developing a schedule.

Your Newborn Needs a Mommie Who:

- Takes naps whenever she can.
- Eats good foods.
- Drinks to thirst.
- Doesn't do housework (except what's absolutely necessary).
- Tries to stay calm and relaxed.
- Isn't entertaining lots of friends.
- Does what she likes most: reading, listening to music, watching movies, talking with friends.
- Nurses frequently.

꩜ 3

Problems, Health, and Special Situations

"Scott was born in the birthing room at the hospital. They laid him on my stomach for a minute, cut the cord, took him over and weighed him, and kind of wiped the goop off. Then they gave him back so I could nurse him right then. I had inverted nipples and I was worried about that. But once he started nursing they came out. They inverted when I wasn't nursing but stayed out when I was. I had no other problems; it all just worked out real well from the beginning."

Don't be overwhelmed by this chapter. Most of the difficulties you encounter in breastfeeding are not serious and will be temporary. The suggestions offered here will help you to correct most of the problems that come up. However, don't hesitate to get further assistance from your physician, midwife, childbirth instructor, lactation consultant, or representatives of La Leche League (see Resources, page 204).

COMMON PROBLEMS

Engorgement

Engorgement is swelling caused by increased fluid and blood in the breast tissue, and/or by the accumulation of milk. The nipples may flatten, making it hard for the baby to grasp them. The breasts become full, hard, painful, and sometimes warm. The condition usually starts about two days after the baby's birth (when your milk starts to come in) but will disappear within two to seven days if properly cared for. Shorter bouts of engorgement may recur due to missed feedings, and it is a common plight among working mothers, particularly when they first return to work.

What to Do:
- Breastfeed as soon as possible after the baby's birth and at frequent intervals (one and a half to three hours during the day; four to five hours at night).
- Use both breasts at each feeding.
- Manually express some milk before the feeding to soften the areola.
- Use warm packs or take a warm shower before feeding. Manually express some milk while you are in the shower.
- Alternating warm and cold water may reduce discomfort between feedings.
- When you miss a feeding, express enough milk to ease the discomfort (more if possible). If you frequently miss feedings, you need to empty your breasts completely in order to maintain your supply. In Chapter Four, we will discuss how much to express while you are at work.
- Plastic breast shields (milk shells or cups) can be worn for short periods; they exert pressure around the nipples to draw out excess milk.

Sore or Cracked Nipples

Tenderness of the nipples is common in breastfeeding, and sometimes the skin breaks (it may or may not bleed). Some pain when the baby first grasps the nipple is normal; persistent pain and cracking should be cared for.

What to Do:
- Make sure the baby is positioned correctly, with her head and body facing your breast. Support her head so that her chin is against your breast and there is no downward pull on the nipple. Make sure the nipple and most of the areola are in the baby's mouth.
- Position the baby with her face, chest, belly, and especially the knees facing you. The knees should touch your belly. This puts the baby's chin in alignment.
- Express some milk before each feeding to soften the nipple and areola.
- Nurse on the breast that is less sore first, with the other nipple exposed to the air. If you are engorged, offer the sorer breast first.
- Feed more frequently (every one and a half to three hours) for shorter periods (ten to fifteen minutes).
- Apply some expressed milk to your nipples and areola, and let it dry there between feedings.
- Air dry your nipples for at least five minutes after each feeding.
- Avoid petroleum-based ointments such as vitamin A and D ointments, baby oil, and Vaseline, because they keep out air. Also, avoid creams containing alcohol, as they dry the skin. Remember, too, that many ointments have a taste which the baby may not like. The La Leche League recommends applying a few drops of your own milk to the nipple, and then allowing it to air dry. If you do decide to use an ointment, apply it sparingly. The La

Leche League suggests ultra-purified, medical-grade anhydrous lanolin, made by Lansinoh.
- Wash with water; avoid using soap.
- Keep your bra and nursing pads dry. If your nipples are so sore that a bra or clothing is painful, try wearing breast shells (with large nipple openings and air holes) or tea strainers in your bra to protect the nipples.
- Pain could be caused by thrush, an oral infection passed back and forth between the baby's mouth and your breast. If you suspect that your baby has this infection, your physician should be contacted, and both your nipples and the baby's mouth will be treated with antifungal medication. You do not need to stop breastfeeding.

Blocked Ducts

These are tender areas or lumps in the breast.

What to Do:
- Begin nursing on the affected side. Empty that breast completely, using manual expression if necessary.
- Massage the area from the base of the breast out toward the nipple.
- Apply warm packs to the area.
- Make sure your bra is not too tight.
- Feed frequently, and alternate the baby's positions to ease the flow of milk from the ducts.
- When you miss a feeding (e.g., at work), make sure you express enough milk manually.
- Avoid sleeping on the affected side.

Mastitis

Mastitis is an infected area in the breast that causes redness, pain, heat, fever, chills, flu-like symptoms, and occasionally nausea and vomiting. It does not usually occur until several weeks after the birth of the baby and is sometimes precipitated by hectic schedules that interfere with complete nursing, a bra that is too tight, or pressure from very large breasts that are not receiving adequate support.

What to Do:
- Rest in bed. Keep the baby in bed with you and enlist the help of others.
- Drink to thirst.
- Use the methods suggested for blocked ducts.
- Continue to nurse from both breasts, beginning with the unaffected side. Then switch to the affected side as soon as your milk lets down.
- Nurse on the affected side frequently.
- Make sure the affected side is completely emptied (use manual expression if necessary).
- Use moist, warm packs to alleviate discomfort. Sometimes ice also helps.
- Bathe your breasts in warm water.
- Contact your physician. If an antibiotic is prescribed, it should be one that is safe for the baby (see "Maternal Illness and Drugs," page 50). A full ten-day course of antibiotics is advised to prevent a relapse.
- Take Ibuprofen for pain and fever at the discretion of you and your practitioner.
- It is not necessary to stop nursing.

Fussy or Colicky Baby

Fussy babies are difficult to comfort and sometimes pull away and cry at the beginning of a feeding. A colicky baby often cries for several hours at the same time every day, with her body tensed and her legs drawn up in pain.

What to Do:
- Change the baby's position frequently, providing new things for her to look at. Walk, rock, swing. Hold her close

to your body. Sometimes the father or grandparent, or anyone besides the mother, can comfort the baby better.

- Check your diet for possible problem foods such as garlic, cabbage, turnips, broccoli, or too much fresh fruit.
- Make sure your milk is letting down. Review the techniques for stimulating let-down (Chapter Two).
- Is milk gushing too fast into the baby's mouth at the beginning of a feeding? This can frustrate the baby and cause her to pull away and cry. Express a little milk before the baby latches on.
- Relax and avoid becoming overtired. The baby senses when you are uptight.
- Make sure the baby is getting enough. See "Insufficient Breastmilk," below.
- The baby may need to be burped frequently. Gently massage her back or tummy.
- The baby may be having a growth spurt, usually at two weeks, four to six weeks, and three months. Nurse frequently to build up your supply.
- The baby may be having a bad day. Give her lots of cuddles. Nurse frequently.
- Try nursing a colicky baby this way: Lie on your back and support your head with pillows. Position the baby stomach-down across your chest and support her head with the palm of your hand. If feeding this way, the baby is less apt to gulp and takes in less air.
- Use a baby carrier that carries the baby upright on your chest.
- Leave your baby in the care of someone you trust and get out for a while.

Insufficient Breastmilk

If the baby is nursing from eight to ten times a day, has six or more wet diapers, and is gaining about a pound a month, she is getting enough milk. (Note: Newborns typically lose 5 percent of their body weight after birth, and up to 10 percent is considered okay as long as no other problems are present.) But most mothers worry at one time or another about whether their baby is getting enough to eat.

What to Do:
- Nurse frequently. Use both breasts at each feeding.
- Make sure the baby takes at least one night feeding. Wake her if necessary.
- If the baby is not a strong suckler, feed her more frequently.
- Make sure your diet is complete and well balanced, and that you are not taking any medications that might be interfering with your supply.
- Get plenty of rest.
- Check your let-down reflex (good indications are a tingling sensation as the milk rushes in, leakage, a spurt of milk from the non-nursing breast, or the sound of baby swallowing rythmically).
- Avoid giving bottles until your supply is well established (after about three weeks). If breastfeeding is going well, you do not need supplements. If it is not going well, supplements will make matters worse; it is better to nurse more often. If you must be away for a feeding, express milk manually to be given in the bottle. Complementary bottles (given after the feeding to "top it off") will also sabotage your milk supply. Solid foods are not necessary until about four to six months of age; if given before, they will reduce the time spent at the breast and your supply will diminish.
- Try the techniques recommended in "Fussy or Colicky Baby."
- Consult your pediatrician to evaluate the baby's weight gain and the quality of your milk.
- Use a feeding tube device (page 52).

Baby Refuses Breast

Sometimes a baby takes a while to get started. She may not latch on right away, and it may take her a number of tries before she gets the hang of nursing. As you try the following techniques, be patient. Sometimes a baby will prefer one breast over the other. This can be caused by a different breast shape, nipple size, or let-down reflex. Occasionally a baby refuses both sides. The return of menstruation sometimes causes the baby to reject the breast for a couple of days at the beginning of the period. It is also possible that the mother has eaten a strong food that the baby simply doesn't like.

What to Do:
- Check the baby's position. Make sure her nose isn't squashed into the breast and blocking breathing.
- Check the baby's nose for mucus that might block breathing during suckling.
- Call your pediatrician if you suspect that the baby is ill, and check her temperature.
- Manually express milk from the refused breast to make grasping easier and to start milk flowing.
- Change the baby to the rejected breast without altering her body position (use a football hold to prop her on your arm so that her body faces the same direction it did on the favorite breast).
- If you have your period, be persistent in your offers to nurse. The baby's rejection is temporary.
- Review your diet for strongly flavored foods the baby might find offensive.
- If refusal of one breast continues despite all these efforts, it is wise to have the breast checked by your physician to rule out specific pathology.

STAYING HEALTHY

During pregnancy your body stores fat and other nutrients in preparation for lactation and to make sure you have a nutritional reserve stashed away for days when you don't eat very well. When you are lactating your baby gets served first, so an inadequate diet will drain your body of nutrients before it goes after your milk and depletes it. It has been shown, however, that when mothers don't get the right nutrition, the volume of milk can decrease. A good, well-balanced diet will ensure a well-fed baby and a healthy you, as well as an adequate supply of milk.

Nursing mothers are often advised to drink to thirst, which ordinarily is not a problem since breastfeeding makes you very thirsty. Watch out, though, when you go back to work. This is a time when mothers start forgetting the need for liquids. To remind you, keep a glass of water or juice beside you at all times. If you don't get enough fluids it probably won't affect the amount of your milk, but you will urinate less, become listless, and in hot weather you may be in danger of dehydration.

You should begin nutritional preparation for breastfeeding during pregnancy or, ideally, before. The Committee on Recommended Dietary Allowances of the Food and Nutrition Board advises that during pregnancy you meet all the RDAs for adult women *plus* an increase in calories (300), protein (30 grams), all vitamins and minerals (various increases), folic acid (100 percent), calcium, phosphorus, and magnesium (50 percent). For lactation, you further increase most of the pregnancy levels of recommended nutrients. You can meet these increases by adding two cups of milk, two ounces of meat or peanut butter, an extra vegetable and extra fruit, a glass of citrus juice, and a slice of whole-wheat bread. If you are a strict vegetarian (no eggs or dairy products), an additional supplement of up to 4 mcg/day of vitamin B_{12} is recommended. (See table of RDAs for lactating women.)

RECOMMENDED DIETARY ALLOWANCES FOR PREGNANT AND LACTATING ADULT WOMEN (1989)*

Nutrient	Adult Pregnant Female	Adult Lactating Female (First six months)	Adult Lactating Female (Second six months)
Protein (g)	60	65	62
Vitamin A (μg)	800	1,300	1,200
Vitamin D (μg)	10	10	10
Vitamin E (mg)	10	12	11
Vitamin K (μg)	65	65	65
Vitamin C (mg)	70	95	90
Thiamine (mg)	1.5	1.6	1.6
Riboflavin (mg)	1.6	1.8	1.7
Niacin (mg)	17	20	20
Vitamin B_6 (mg)	2.2	2.1	2.1
Folate (μg)	400	280	260
Vitamin B_{12} (μg)	2.2	2.6	2.6
Calcium (mg)	1,200	1,200	1,200
Phosphorus (mg)	1,200	1,200	1,200
Magnesium (mg)	300	355	340
Iron (mg)	30	15	15
Zinc (mg)	15	19	16
Iodine (μg)	175	200	200
Selenium (μg)	65	75	75

*Recommended Dietary Allowances, National Research Council, National Academy of Sciences, Washington, D.C.

It is not wise to diet during lactation, and as mentioned before, most women find they don't need to. The extra calories required to produce breastmilk (maybe about five hundred) will constitute a natural weight-loss program. If you are trying to lose weight, you can increase the nutrients you take in without increasing the calories one bit by choosing foods carefully and avoiding empty calories (foods that have calories but provide few nutrients). The additional calories needed for producing milk can be met by fat stores accumulated during pregnancy (read: bye-bye, fat). When you have reached your prepregnancy weight, you should increase your caloric intake. Any additional weight loss should be very gradual—no more than one pound per week (safer yet is one pound every two weeks).

Foods to Avoid

Some infants get very crabby about certain foods. Garlic, cabbage, turnips, broccoli, beans, rhubarb, apricots, and prunes have been associated with gassy, colicky periods in some babies. A heavy dose of melons and fresh fruits could be the culprit in some cases of colic and diarrhea, as could cow's milk, chocolate, and wheat products.

Hey wait! What's left to eat? Don't worry. Your baby will not react to all of these foods and may not have trouble with any of them. If you suspect a particular food, however, keep track of when you eat it and when the colic appears. If you identify a connection, avoid the offender. If you cannot identify the food, eliminate the following items from your diet in this order: first, cow's milk; second, citrus fruit; third, wheat products; fourth, chocolate. Then observe if and when your baby's reaction is relieved.

If your family has a history of allergies, you should avoid allergens to which you and any members of your family are sensitive.

In one report, coffee was included as a drug rather than

a food, and there were studies cited in which 1 percent of the caffeine ingested by the mother appeared in her milk. Caffeine received this way by the infant reaches a danger level when the mother drinks about twenty cups per day. However, much lower levels have been associated with fussy babies.

Maternal Illness and Drugs

What if you get sick? With few exceptions, you can nurse your baby, even when you are sick (see Chapter One, "When Not to Breastfeed"). However, an illness or infection might affect your milk supply. Contact your doctor right away if you become ill, and make sure he or she knows you are breastfeeding in case antibiotics or other medications are necessary.

Almost all drugs present in your blood will enter your milk to some degree. Researchers are still a long way from any definitive conclusions about maternal drugs because their effect on the infant depends on numerous factors. Even the aspirin question is not completely settled, and women requiring a lot of aspirin therapy are advised to investigate an alternative drug. Drugs vary in their characteristics, how they are dissolved and transported, and how they are absorbed, detoxified, and excreted by the baby. The most important considerations are: (1) Is the drug one that could be safely given to the infant directly? (2) If so, what would be the risks? (3) What is a safe dosage? (4) Do the benefits of breastfeeding outweigh the risks of the drug?

When you need medication, your physician should select a drug that will appear in the least amount in the milk and carries the least risk to the baby. Dosages can be scheduled to minimize the amount in the milk (e.g., right after a feeding). While you are taking medication, watch your baby for any changes such as sleeping more, feeding less than usual, fussiness, or a rash. Dark stools (caused by blood) have been associated with aspirin.

CESAREAN BIRTH

If you know in advance that you are going to have a cesarean section, you will have some time to prepare yourself emotionally and physically, and you can also make arrangements and decisions to facilitate the earliest possible contact with your baby for breastfeeding. If, however, your cesarean is unplanned, it can be more traumatic and is probably a result of a medical emergency that changes the circumstances following birth.

If you feel well enough after a cesarean birth, and depending on the type of anesthesia that was used, you may be able to nurse within the first twelve hours. Mothers have nursed within the first hour. If you have regional anesthesia, you will be awake and can possibly nurse as soon as you and the baby are stabilized. At first you will need lots of help in finding a comfortable position. If you have had a spinal anesthetic requiring you to remain flat for a while after birth, the best position for nursing is on your side with the baby supported against you. In some cases, the medication given to the mother during birth can depress the baby and weaken the suckling response. After birth you will probably need pain medication, which is safe provided the drugs are carefully chosen. The pain medications prescribed should be easily excreted by you and the baby and are best administered immediately after a feeding to allow the drug to peak before the next feeding.

If the newborn needs to be cared for in a special-care nursery, the opportunity to nurse will be delayed, and this will delay the beginning of lactation. Pumping or hand expression of milk will help to stimulate your supply until your baby begins nursing regularly.

You will need a lot of rest and the support of those around you both in the hospital and when you get home. Though it may present more difficulties at first, cesarean birth in no way precludes breastfeeding your baby. (See Resources for organizations that offer information and support to ce-sarean mothers.)

PREMATURE BIRTH

If your baby is born prematurely (before thirty-seven weeks of gestation) or has a low birthweight (under five pounds, eight ounces), she may initially be cared for in a special-care nursery. The breastmilk you supply at this stage will be via bottle or gavage tube with milk you have ex-pressed. Any milk you give is important, and expression of colostrum to be given to your baby supplies valuable antibod-ies. Sometimes larger premature infants can be weaned from the incubator and tried on the breast within twenty-four hours. Their suckling reflexes may be poor at first, but they can get some colostrum this way as well as provide brief stim-ulation of the breast. Until your baby is strong and mature enough to suckle vigorously, you can maintain your supply by manual expression and pumping. This takes patience and de-termination, and in some circumstances emotional or geo-graphical problems make this routine too difficult.

How soon your baby can be nipple fed or breastfed de-pends on her size and the state of her health. Until the suck-ling reflex is well established, premature babies are usually fed using a combination of the gavage tube, the bottle, and the breast. Even if the mother has an adequate supply, these in-fants are not yet strong enough to get all the nutrition they need from the breast. A feeding tube device, which supplies supplement to the baby through a tube while she nurses at the breast, makes it possible for the baby to receive enough nourishment while stimulating the mother's milk production. This method can also prevent the difficult transition bottle-fed premature babies sometimes experience when they try to adapt to the breast.

You will need lots of support and information as you

make decisions and plan for the care of a baby born too soon or too small. *The Premature Baby Book* by Helen Harrison (St. Martin's Press) is an excellent guidebook, with a comprehensive appendix listing books, organizations, and resources to assist families with premature infants.

4

Meals on Wheels

"I had to be at work at eight o'clock, and I got off at about five. Not real strict hours—if I was a little late, or if I had to leave, no problem. I nursed Eric on my lunch hour until he was six months old, so every day at noon I went over to the babysitter's and nursed him. Not always right at noon—the sitter would call me and tell me when he was hungry. He was eight minutes away. I ate at my desk whenever I was hungry. Usually it took about an hour and twenty minutes to nurse him, because I didn't like to leave right after he was done—a lot of times he'd fall asleep, so I'd wait for him to get the other side. And it was great just to hold him during the day; it was a nice break. When he was real small and taking more feedings, I pumped in the morning and in the afternoon.

"I pumped in the women's bathroom in the stall. I expressed about four to five ounces at one *time. I used a jar, put it into my little sack and stuck it in the refrigerator at work.*

"I felt like everybody thought I was weird. Because at that time there were four girls there working in the same office, and they were all going to have babies. None of them expressed the desire to nurse at all, much less hassling with that during the day. They thought it was a big pain. And it was, it wasn't easy. It was hard to get the schedule going at first. But I thought that was the best thing for him and I wanted to do it as long as I could—give him everything that I thought was healthier for him.

"I did this until Eric was six months old. Then he started eating a little bit of cereal, and that cut down on the milk he wanted. For maybe a month I pumped once a day, during noon or in the afternoon. He did have some supplemental formula, but I fed him in the morning before I left, and he had a bottle at noon that was frozen [breastmilk] from the day before. Then right when I got home from work I nursed him, and then before he went to bed, and usually in the middle of the night.

"I didn't care what people thought. I knew what I was doing was right. It was the best thing for Eric. I liked being close to him. It was better for his health, and it made me feel better. I always felt a little bit healthier when I was breastfeeding.

"I feel closer to Eric than I would if I hadn't breastfed. I felt pretty darn guilty when I went back; the first couple of weeks, it was terrible. I wanted to be with him. Breastfeeding really helped.

"I think if women are going to go back to work, they ought to try to breastfeed for as long as they can. It's not easy, but it's every bit worth it. It

*made me feel like he still needed me. It made me
feel good to still be needed even though I wasn't
with him all day. I was still giving him something
from me even though I wasn't right there."*

Figuring out how your baby will be fed during the
hours you are at work is the first step in planning your work-
ing/breastfeeding agenda. Unless you work at home or in a
flexible job that allows you to be available for all of your
baby's meals, you will need to devise a strategy for the feedings you miss. When you miss a feeding, your breasts need to
be emptied to maintain your supply. As your baby grows and
demands more, the amount you need to express at work increases. If you don't keep pace this way, your supply may
gradually diminish and your baby may be weaned earlier than
you wish. Many mothers express and save their breastmilk
for the next day's feedings; some who travel discard the expressed milk and provide formula for their babies during
working hours. A few traveling women manage to take their
babies along, or store expressed milk until they get home.
And there are a number of women who do little or no pumping; they breastfeed during the hours they are at home and
provide formula for missed feedings. As will be discussed
later, this last technique requires a well-established milk
supply.

With most of these choices, you will have to become a
bit of an expert at hand expressing or pumping breastmilk,
and you will need to find both the time and a place in which
to do it. Once you are back on the job, your time will be limited and you will probably feel anxious and self-conscious the
first few times you slip off to pump. The more efficient your
pumping techniques become, the less inconvenient will be
this brief excursion away from your desk or job assignment.

You can express the milk from your breasts manually or
with the help of a breast pump. Women who choose the manual method do so because it's simpler (once you learn to do

it), requires no extra equipment except what is used for containing and storage, and for them, it is more sanitary and comfortable. Sometimes pumps cause nipple soreness or red "ring around the nipple." For others, manual expression is difficult, feels awkward, or simply does not produce the quantity of milk removed by a pump. It is a good idea to experiment with both methods before you return to work. Practice until you are skilled in the technique that works best for you. Remember that the principle of the let-down reflex is the same whether you are nursing or pumping.

"The first several days I manually expressed my milk, my hands and breasts were sore. But it didn't take long, and I was a real pro," says Carolyn F., a property manager who returned to work when her son was two months old and nursed him for seventeen months. "Within one week I was expressing five ounces two times a day. As my baby ate more, I expressed more. After two months I was expressing sixteen ounces—eight ounces two times a day—taking fifteen to twenty minutes each time."

"My biggest problem was letting down," says Emily D., who breastfed her daughter for ten months while working as an office supervisor for a lumber manufacturer. "And getting relaxed enough and trying not to think about other things so it would happen. I tried to think about holding Dawn and having her there and that helped. But then when I was sitting there in the rest room talking to myself people thought I was crazy." Emily used a combination technique—the pump first, to get the flow going, followed by manual expression. For her, manual expression produced more milk.

Kathy M., a schoolteacher, takes about fifteen minutes of her lunch hour to express milk. "I want to have some time to sit and eat lunch and get ready to go before the kids come back in." Kathy laughs about the day a student wandered into the teacher's lounge while she was pumping her milk. "Here I was, leaned over the sink running warm water over my hands [to help the let-down] when she came in. So I said, nonchalantly, 'Well, I think I'll just wash these dishes.' I got the soap out and started rinsing the dishes. I had the breast pump under my sweater, and she would really have had to look to notice that there was anything there, but all the other teachers were cracking up."

How to Express Manually

- Wash your hands thoroughly.
- Find a place that is warm, comfortable, and private. Take several deep breaths and concentrate on letting your shoulders and body go limp. Think of your wonderful baby.
- Begin by massaging or stroking your breasts in a downward motion toward the nipples. (See illustration below.) You can cup your breast with your hands and slide your hands forward, or you can massage with your fingertips using small circular motions. Rotate the massage around the entire breast.

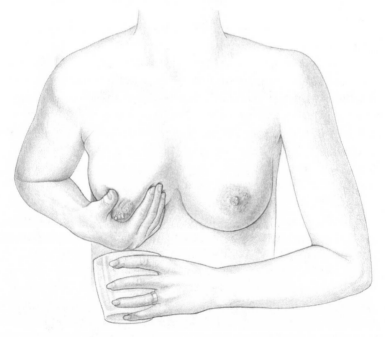

- Position your hand with the thumb on top near the edge of the areola and one or two fingers supporting underneath. Lean forward to let gravity assist with the milk flow. (See illustration below.)
- Press your thumb and fingers against the chest wall, then release as your fingers compress just behind the outer edge of the areola. This should be done rhythmically, like the baby's suckling. Rotate the position of your hand so other milk reservoirs are drained. (See illustrations, page 60.)
- Don't pull or squeeze.
- The spray will resemble the medium setting on the spray bottle for houseplants. Or it may drip and spray.
- Change hands, alternating positions: left hand/left breast; right hand/left breast; right hand/right breast; left hand/right breast.

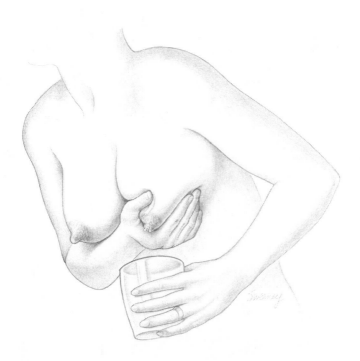

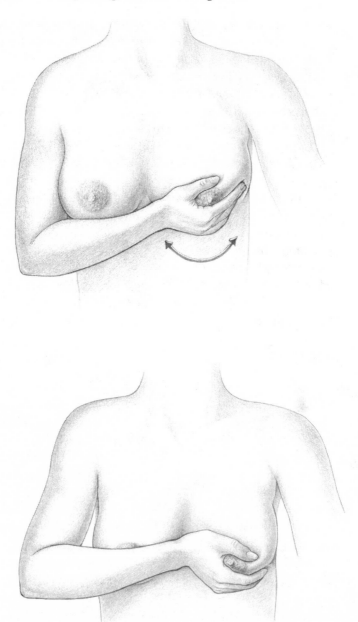

• You can express one side completely, then switch to the other. Or you can switch back and forth. As long as both breasts are emptied, your method will be a matter of preference, speed, and comfort.

Breast Pumps

There are three categories of breast pumps: manual, electrical, and battery-operated, with a wide variety of models and manufacturers. All of them create a vacuum (negative pressure), which draws the milk out of the breast and into a bottle or container. Cylinder pumps are constructed with an inner and outer cylinder; the inner cylinder serves as the piston drawing milk into the outer cylinder. Other manual pumps are designed with a separate pump mechanisms, and the milk is extracted into an attached bottle. "Bicycle horn" pumps are not recommended, because the sucking action is not very good and the pump cannot be sterilized. Electrical and battery-operated pumps operate on the same principles, but the pumping is done for you. Many women prefer electrical pumps because they are faster and, for some, easier. However, electrical pumps are more expensive (costing as much as $700).

Some breast pumps come with adaptors that fit inside the flange (the part that you press against your breast) to adjust for varying nipple sizes. "It took me quite a while to express at first," says Lisa T. "I was using the smaller nipple adaptor, thinking that my nipple was small enough for it. What I ended up doing was changing to the bigger one out of frustration one day, and the bigger one was what I needed to get enough suction and to cover enough of the areola. I think I was plugging up half of my milk ducts. Once I changed, there was no problem."

As with manual expression, it is important to empty both breasts. You may want to complete one side before starting the other, or switch back and forth if your nipples become sore from the pulling action of the pump. Some electrical pumps offer an attachment that allows you to pump from both breasts at the same time. This makes pumping faster and avoids leakage that you sometimes get from the breast that isn't being pumped.

If your physician prescribes a breast pump for you while you are in the hospital, all or part of the cost may be covered by your health insurance. Some insurance companies routinely pay for breast pumps without a doctor's prescription. Contact your insurance company before your baby is born to find out if your policy covers a breast pump and if you will need a prescription or letter from your physician. To obtain insurance coverage, the prescription must be written in your baby's name, not yours. (For problems or questions regarding insurance, contact the insurance commission in your state.)

Some of the more expensive electrical pumps can be rented and the cost shared with other mothers. Ann M., a nurse, used the hospital's electrical pump for all of her expressing, but this kind of convenience is not likely to be found except in health-care centers. Realistically, you will probably buy a hand pump of your own, and for that reason you need to be as choosy as you can. It's a good idea to shop around before your baby is born—among drug stores, department stores, and baby shops. Then if you don't find what you want, you will have time to order it.

Sometimes pumps come in kits, ceremoniously labeled "breast feeding systems," with nipples, covers, nipple adaptors, spare parts, cleaning brush, freezer bags, and self-adhesive tags for labeling the date on the milk. You may not need all of the items in the kit, and you may be able to put together your own kit for less money. For example, you can make your own tags with adhesive tape and provide your own storage containers. When you purchase a pump make sure you will be able to buy spare parts separately in case you lose a part or one needs to be replaced. With some pumps, the gaskets wear out frequently.

It is important to read and carefully follow the instructions on the pump. The best way to learn how to use a pump is to have someone show you. Be sure you observe the manufacturer's instructions for cleaning the pump and its parts.

A good pump can make the difference between a smooth, satisfying workday milk expression and one that is a hassle you could do without. Choose your pump carefully. Also, some pumps are a bit tight at first, and it takes a couple of weeks before the rubber gaskets are worn in and move with ease.

The following are guidelines to help you make your selection.

Selecting a Breast Pump

A good breast pump should . . .

- Empty the breasts completely in a reasonably short period of time (about twenty minutes).
- Be easy to clean.
- Be portable.
- Provide intermittent pressure (rather than continuous, which can bruise or rupture the breast).
- Provide enough pressure to extract milk efficiently.
- Have features to stimulate let-down and milk flow:
  1. flare of the nipple cup is wide and deep
  2. shank of the nipple cup is long and wide enough for nipple distention
  3. adaptors for different nipple sizes
  4. pump flange nipple insert is about the width of your index finger
- Have a collection area that is see-through so you can measure the amount of milk pumped.
- Be easy to use (If you are right-handed, is the pump awkward when you use your left hand? If so, you may not empty one breast as well).
- Be constructed so milk does not spray into bulb if it is the bulb type (makes it hard to clean).
- Have an outer cylinder or collection vessel that converts to a bottle (optional).

Tips on Using a Hand Pump

- Read the instructions.
- Wash or sterilize the pump parts. (Sterilization is recommended for babies under one month of age or babies who are ill.)
- Find a relaxing position in a quiet spot. Use breast massage, a warm cloth, and relaxation techniques (deep breathing, imagining your baby, looking at your baby's picture).
- Select the nipple adaptor that fits your nipple closely yet allows the nipple to slip into the opening. Your nipple should be centered in the opening.
- When you are learning, try pumping after a feeding, when your milk is already flowing.
- Begin by pushing and pulling the plunger gently and slowly. It will take practice to establish a steady stream of milk.
- Switching to the second breast after a few minutes on the first breast can take advantage of the let-down stimulated on the second breast by the pumping of the first. Then switch back again to completely empty each breast. Or you can completely empty the first breast before switching.

Collecting and Storing Your Milk

Up until a few years ago, experts recommended that you cool your expressed milk immediately. Now, recent research has found that breast milk contains certain bacteria-fighting properties, and can be stored at room temperature for a short time. New recommendations give you a choice: If you refrigerate the milk immediately, you can save it for up to five days. Or, you can keep it at room temperature for six to ten hours, after which you must discard it. Colostrum can be kept at room temperature for twelve to twenty-four hours. These guidelines are outlined in *The Breastfeeding Answer Book* by La Leche League International. There are other sources that recommend a shorter storage time for refrigerated milk. The Human Milk Banking Association of North America, Inc., recommends freezing milk that is not used within forty-eight hours. Its 1993 guidelines state: "A general rule to remember is that the longer milk is stored and the more 'processing' it undergoes, the more it loses in nutrient and immunologic content." If you do decide to cool your milk, you can also use an insulated thermos or cooler with ice or cool packs ("blue ice"). Or, you can splurge on a natty carrying case, designed specifically for this purpose, with a storage compartment and place for your pump.

For storage, plastic containers are best, and if the milk will be frozen, either glass or hard plastic is okay. If you are adding milk to a supply already in storage, it is best to express the milk in a separate clean container, cool the milk, and then add it to the supply. This keeps the new milk from warming the stored batch. Specially designed plastic milk storage bags are okay, too, but be sure to follow the directions for sealing and opening the bags, to avoid contamination.

Freeze your milk in one-feeding amounts. Most experts discourage "layering"—adding fresh milk to frozen—because the fresh milk can thaw the top portion of the frozen. However, if you cool the fresh milk first, it can be safely added to the frozen. ALWAYS LABEL YOUR MILK WITH THE DATE.

The La Leche League guidelines for freezing breast milk are as follows:

- Two weeks in a freezer compartment inside the refrigerator;
- Three to four months in a self-contained freezer compartment of a refrigerator;
- Six months or longer in a separate deep freeze held at constant 0°F.

Thaw milk under cool running water, gradually heating the water to bring the milk to room temperature. Or, thaw the container in a pan of water that has been heated to lukewarm on the stove, but do not thaw a container of milk directly on the stove. DO NOT THAW FROZEN MILK IN A MICROWAVE. Microwaves not only thaw unevenly, but the higher temperatures in the microwave destroy nutrients.

Do not refreeze milk. Milk left in the feeding container should be discarded. If milk has been thawed but not warmed yet, you can save it in the refrigerator for up to twenty-four hours.

Whether or not you sterilize bottles and containers is a matter you may want to discuss with your health-care provider. Many doctors no longer recommend boiling equipment; hot soapy water or a dishwasher are considered sufficient for cleaning your supplies as long as you clean them thoroughly. If you do decide to sterilize, wash and rinse the containers and place them in a pan of cold water. Put the lid on the pan and bring the water to a boil. Boil for five minutes and then turn off the heat. Once you have sterilized the containers, don't touch the insides. Follow your manufacturer's instructions for sterilizing your breast pump.

Now, let's return to the workplace, where we find ourselves hunting for a refrigerator. There is bound to be one somewhere in most businesses. If there is an employee lounge or break room, it's easy, once you get over the initial self-consciousness of plunking your breastmilk down next to someone's salami sandwich. If everyone knows what you are doing, and your milk is clearly labeled, no one will bother it and your little containers will become part of the scenery. Or you can use a lunch box or brown bag and no one will even know what's inside.

If there isn't an employee refrigerator, you may have to seek one out. Is there a kitchen or commissary on the premises? Speak with your supervisor and inquire about the procedure to follow in order to obtain permission to use the refrigerator. Explain that you will be making, at the most, three quick trips (two for delivery and one for pickup at the end of the day). This could hardly cause much disruption.

How Long Should It Take to Express?

These are optimum times, not meant to place stopwatch pressure on you, but rather to show how expression can be fit into a work break. Many women experience difficulties with pumping and will need more time than is suggested here. The more experienced you become, the faster you will be. At first, allow an extra five or ten minutes, especially if you are expressing by hand, because proficiency with manual expression takes a bit longer to attain. If you use an electrical pump, follow the time guide for manual expression.

Hint: If you work five days a week, the amount you pump may decrease on days four and five.

Manually

- Preparation (wash hands, undo clothing and bra, massage breasts and position hand): about five minutes.
- Express milk: about ten minutes.
- Replace clothing and store milk: about five minutes.

Total time: about twenty minutes.

Breast Pump

- Preparation (wash hands, assemble pump, undo clothing and bra, massage breasts, position pump): about five minutes.
- Pump milk and place in storage container: about twenty minutes.
- Replace clothing, rinse pump: about five minutes.

Total time: about thirty minutes.

MANUAL AND BATTERY PUMPS

Name	Description
Ameda/Egnell	**Manual** One hand; compact enough to fit in a purse; Mom controls cycling and suction; pump directly into a freezer bag.
Ameda/Egnell	**Cylinder**
Comfort Plus Omron Healthcare, Inc.	**Manual** Angled breast flange for comfortable lactation; pump easily converts to storage/nurser bottle after expression.

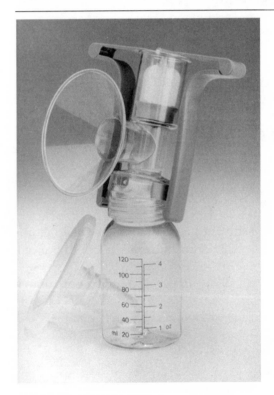

Ameda/Egnell
Manual Breast Pump

Approx. Cost	To order, or for more information
$29.50	Ameda/Egnell 755 Industrial Drive Cary, IL 60013-1993 800-323-8750
$25.00	same as manual
$12.00	Omron Healthcare, Inc. Juvenile Division 300 Lakeview Parkway Vernon Hills, IL 60061 800-922-2959

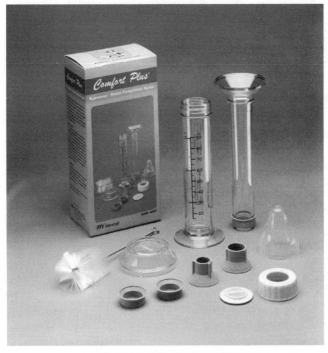

Comfort Plus Cylinder Breast Pump

MANUAL AND BATTERY PUMPS

Name	Description
MagMag Advanced Omron Healthcare, Inc.	**Battery/AC adaptable** Lightweight and portable; added stability with motor at base; unique collection and storage system allows refrigerating/freezing, warming, and feeding from the same container; suction control button and convenient suction release button; chime sounds if the motor ever needs flushing.
Omron Healthcare, Inc.	**Travel Pack** Therm O Tote or Fanny Pack Plus (each sold separately).
Gentle Expressions	**Battery/AC adaptable** Portable; battery operated/AC adaptable; suction comfort control valves; intermittent suction release; one hand operation.
Gentle Expressions	**Travel Pack** includes pump

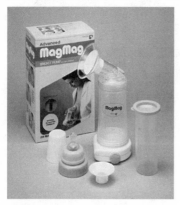

MagMag Advanced Battery/AC
Adaptable Breast Pump

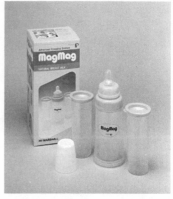

MagMag Advanced Freezing
System

Approx. Cost	To order, or for more information
$34.50	same as manual
$6.50 $7.15	same as manual
$44.95	The Lumiscope Company, Inc. 400 Raritan Center Parkway Edison, NJ 08837 800-221-5747
$79.95	same as battery/AC adaptable

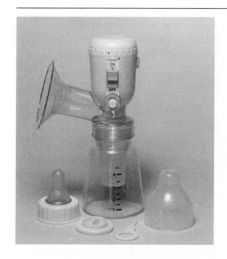

Gentle Expressions Battery/AC
Adaptable Breast Pump
(LUMISCOPE)

MANUAL AND BATTERY PUMPS

Name	Description
Gerber	**Cylinder** Comes with a cleaning brush and breastfeeding guide.
Gerber	**Battery/Electric** Express breast milk easily and comfortably into nurser; easy feeding and storage; finger-tip vacuum control; soft silicone funnel conforms to mother's shape and size.
Loyd-B	**Manual** Easy to use; does not require constant use of both hands; does not need frequent emptying.
SpringExpress	**Manual** Upgradeable to double pumping with Medela Lactina or Classic Electric Breastpumps with adapter kit; automatic cycling which imitates your baby's nursing action; adjustable vacuum within safe levels for individual comfort.

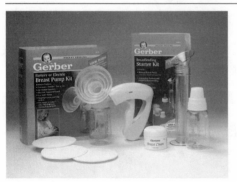

Gerber Battery/Electric Breast Pump and Gerber Cylinder Breast Pump and Starter Kit

Approx. Cost	To order, or for more information
$13.97	available at Target, Walmart, or Toys ' Я' Us Gerber Products Company 445 State Street Fremont, MI 49413-0001 800-443-7237
$45.97	same as cylinder
$39.95	Lopuco, Ltd. 1615 Old Annapolis Road Woodbine, MD 21797 800-634-7867
$27.85	Medela, Inc. P.O. Box 660 McHenry, IL 60051-0660 800-835-5968

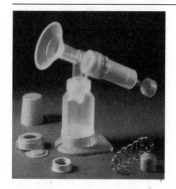

Spring Express Manual Breast Pump
(MEDELA)

ELECTRIC PUMPS

Name	Description
Ameda/Egnell Hygiene Kit	No outside air is vented through collected milk; tubing never needs cleaning; can easily convert to a manual pump.
Ameda/Egnell Elite	Infinite range of safe cycles and suction levels; adjust each suction cycle independently of each other; may pump directly into any collection bottles or freezer bags; features whisper-quiet operations; lightweight; integrated rechargeable battery model also available.
Nurture III	Capable of double pumping; portable; adjustable to your suction and cycle time needs.

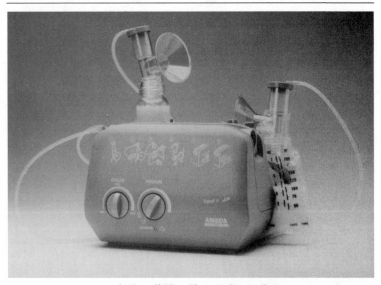

Ameda/Egnell Elite Electric Breast Pump

Approx. Cost	To order, or for more information
$47.25	Ameda/Egnell 755 Industrial Drive Cary, IL 60013-1993 800-323-8750
$650	same as Hygiene Kit
$110	Bailey Medical Engineering 2020 11th Street Los Osos, CA 93402 805-528-5781

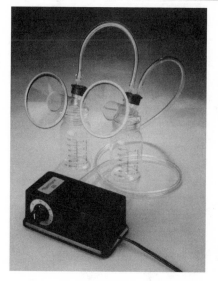

Nurture III Electric Breast Pump
(BAILEY MEDICAL ENGINEERING)

ELECTRIC PUMPS

Name	Description
Mini Electric Medela, Inc.	AC/DC or manual operation; portable; automatically imitates your baby's nursing pattern.
Pump In Style Medela, Inc.	Portable; autocycling; single and double pumping; adjustable vacuum; includes travel bag; operates on battery or vehicle cigarette lighter.
Lactina Select Medela, Inc.	Adjustable pumping speed; adjustable vacuum; automatic sucking action; includes carrying case.

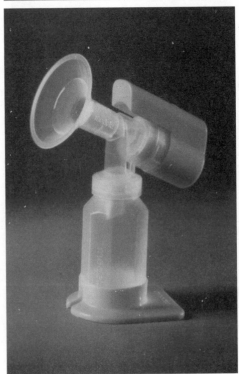

Medela Mini Electric/
Battery Breast Pump

Approx. Cost	To order, or for more information
$86.60	Medela, Inc. P.O. Box 660 McHenry, IL 60051-0660 800-835-5968
$198	same as Mini Electric
$650	same as Mini Electric

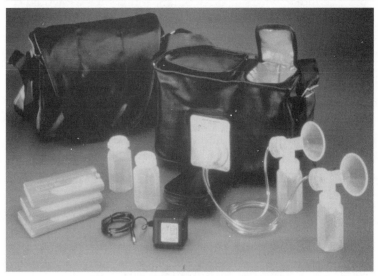

Medela Pump in Style Electric Breast Pump

Where to Pump Your Milk

Before you go back to work, decide where you can go to get the privacy you will need to pump or express. This may necessitate a reconnaissance mission to the office or workplace; you may think you know the premises, but remember that when you left there you weren't looking for places to pump your milk. Also, you should take this time to discuss with your supervisor (if you haven't already) your plans for breastfeeding and working, and explain what your procedure will be.

Christine H., who works for the district court, established this routine: "On Mondays I fed Adam before I went to work, and then usually I would need to pump at around ten-thirty. I was real fortunate because I had a very supportive boss, the judge, who's also a woman. Sometimes we would recess court at about ten-thirty and I could pump then. If I didn't have enough time to pump everything I needed, I could do enough to relieve the discomfort and finish up later. On other days, I would pump in the morning, at about ten-thirty, and again in the afternoon, at about two-thirty. I usually did it in my office because I could lock the door, and there's a bathroom close by. So it worked out real slick, and then we had a refrigerator in the office, so I could keep the milk there. On Monday I'd pump the milk that Adam would be using on Tuesday, and so forth. When I was in court, sometimes I would just pop into the judge's chambers and close the door. I was lucky to have a boss like that."

Look for a setting that is private, warm, and has few potential distractions. You should have a place to sit, or at least stand, comfortably. You'll need a place to put your supplies while you're pumping, and it helps to have a sink nearby. Naturally the ideal place is a quiet lounge with a comfy sofa, clean lavatories, and a refrigerator. Or better still, your own office. However, what most woman find is much less than ideal, and it may take some creativity and imagination before you find the pumping corner that is right for you. Unfortunately, a lot of women get stuck expressing milk in the rest room. This an be okay, as long as it's clean. Some women even like it there.

"The second day I was in the bathroom," says Joan S., a schoolteacher, "one of the gals came in and knocked on the door and said, 'Joan, you don't have to sit in the bathroom all by yourself. Come on into the teachers' room—we promise we won't gawk.' So I've been pumping in there. But I think I might be more successful if I had more privacy. You have to be able to relax. When I was in the bathroom there wasn't anyplace to sit except the john, so I sat there and sort of rested my head on the sink and just let myself relax totally. I got more milk then, versus when I sit in the teachers' room and there are lots of things going on. I'm chatting and not really concentrating on what I'm doing. Alone, I concentrate on relaxing, let my shoulders go limp, take deep breaths, and think about a nice, even flow of milk—and away it comes!"

Popular places for pumping are storage closets, locker rooms, lounges, conference rooms, or an office borrowed from someone else. If your work is outside, you can use your car or a friend's car. When traveling or working on the move, use the rest-room on the airplane, or pop into a department store and borrow a dressing room (you'll get the best reception, if any, in the infants or maternity departments).

In case your place of employment has only one break area, and everyone uses it, you may be able to arrange to take your break at a different time. In workplaces where pumping sites are hard to find, you will need the support of your supervisor and coworkers to come up with a creative solution. That support may not be there. If the logistics of working and breastfeeding become so difficult that they interfere with your enjoyment of both your job and your mothering, you may need to reconsider. If you can change jobs, fine. But this is unrealistic for most women. What *is* realistic is to remind yourself that you tried, that the odds were too stacked against you, and that a mother who comes home frustrated and overstressed is not what your baby needs, breastmilk or not.

Christine H., whose job as a court investigator necessitated interviews with felons in the penitentiary, pumped for three months before she decided she had to give it up.

"The reason I finally had to quit was that my work load was increasing, I was working a lot of hours, and I couldn't fit everything in. I was trying to do everything, like a supermom. For instance, on a day when I had to go to the penitentiary to interview someone, I'd try to plan it for 1:30, hoping that I'd be done in time to get back to the office to pump. But sometimes it wouldn't work that way. I'd get engorged, and when the let-down reflex went, it went! And the jail and the penitentiary were not good places for this. I just wasn't always somewhere I could pump. And I let myself get strung out a little bit. In order to do more work, and to fit more work into smaller periods of time so I'd be able to pump, I was neglecting to do things like eat lunch, drink all the fluids I needed, and that complicated things.

"So I started supplementing Adam with formula—and I would breastfeed in the morning, feed him when I picked him up at night, and again when he went to bed. In between he got formula. I had to work into that gradually—first I cut down to pumping once a day and eventually not at all. About two months later I quit breastfeeding completely.

"It was awful when I quit. I wasn't at all ready to give it up. I cried a lot. But I just couldn't keep up—it was more than I could do. I had to be realistic. Had my situation been a little different, not quite so hectic, I would have liked to have done it for a few more months."

When to Pump

The amount you pump depends on your baby's age and consumption, your work schedule, and how much you are able to express each time. Most women who work an eight-hour day find that by pumping twice a day, at about the same time the baby would normally feed, they can maintain their supply and also provide most of the milk for the next day's feedings. (On days off, you nurse full time.) If you use both morning breaks and afternoon breaks, as well as part of your lunch hour, you'll be doing plenty of pumping and should have little problem with either engorgement or diminishing supply. Women working part time (a four-hour day) may need to pump once while they are away from the baby. While traveling, try to pump at about the same time your baby ordinarily feeds, including during the night, if possible.

Remember, you need to empty the breasts completely if time permits. Also, breastfeed your baby as close as possible to the time you leave for work and as soon as possible when you return, and nurse as long as you can for all the feedings at home. Conscientious expression will work to keep up your supply but is simply not as effective as the baby's suckling for stimulating the milk-producing hormones. Avoid pumping when your baby is around to do the job. If you don't have enough breastmilk for the next day's feedings, plan to supplement with formula tomorrow and let your baby nurse today.

With a forty-five-minute drive to work, Tina P. found that she was simply too tired to get up in the morning to pump. Instead, she pumped during her lunch hour and again as soon as she got home, about three to four ounces each time. This method did not produce quite enough next-day milk for her three-month-old son, Keith, so the sitter gave him formula for one of the feedings. (Sometimes the sitter was able to give Keith a small snack of juice to delay his second feeding until Tina arrived to nurse him.) Tina also gave Keith a small amount of rice cereal mixed with her breastmilk, poured right from the pump. "We just thought he was hungry," she said, adding that he tolerated the formula and the solid food quite well.

What concerns Tina most is supply and demand. "I need to keep pumping, and if I don't pump at noon, then the next day I don't have enough milk." However, by staying relaxed and flexible, she is able to compensate for minor disruptions. For example, one Friday she was unable to pump at noon, but she caught up by nursing all weekend at home, giving no supplements, and expressing the surplus after feedings. By Monday her supply was back up and she had stockpiled an extra five ounces of milk.

Working and breastfeeding is time-consuming. Many will be the days when you're in pumping while everyone else is out lunching. For this, you deserve daily pats on the back, which you should give to yourself if no one else does. Be sure to save enough time to eat a nourishing lunch, or bring one from home, and pack goodies for nibbling during your pumping breaks. And keep a glass of water or juice nearby in case you are thirsty.

Drinking water about an hour before expressing milk "really helps," says Tina P. "When I didn't drink my liquids an hour before, I didn't get as much milk."

Expressing Your Milk

- Find a quiet, clean place where you can sit or stand comfortably.
- Wash your hands.
- Have containers and supplies within reach.
- Place paper towels or a cloth on your lap to catch spills.
- Relax, take several deep breaths, and lean forward.
- Massage your breasts.
- Pump or hand express your milk. Empty one breast, then move to the other, massaging it before you begin. Or you can switch back and forth between breasts.
- Chill or freeze milk immediately.

Freezing and Thawing Breastmilk

- Freeze in clean or sterile containers, in one-feeding amounts.
- Do not fill container to the top. Allow room for expansion as the milk freezes.
- Or freeze in clean ice cube trays. One cube equals

about one ounce. Once frozen, remove cubes and store them in plastic freezer bags.

- *Always label milk with the date.*
- Frozen milk can be stored for three to four months at zero degrees Fahrenheit (in a two-door refrigerator); about two weeks in the freezer compartment of a one-door refrigerator; six months longer in the bottom of a deep-freeze. Store at the back of the freezer compartment.
- To thaw, place container under cold water, then gradually warm the water. If desired, heat to body temperature in a pan of warm water.
- *Do not boil breastmilk.*
- *Never heat breastmilk in a microwave oven.*
- Frozen milk should be used within four hours (like formula) once it is thawed.
- The milk may separate, but that's okay.
- *Never refreeze breastmilk.*
- You can add more milk to a partially filled container. Chill the new milk in the refrigerator first before adding to the frozen milk (otherwise, it might cause the frozen milk to thaw at the top). The milk will look layered, but you can shake it gently to mix it. *After a feeding, do not save any leftover thawed milk. Discard it.*

Brown Baggin'

As a presentence investigator for the district court, Christine H. divides her time among her office, the penitentiary, and the courtroom. She returned to work when her son was six weeks old and continued breastfeeding until he was six months old. Christine pumped milk once in the morning and once in the afternoon, storing it in bottles in a refrigerator at the office.

"People teased me because I had this briefcase and I looked so businesslike going into the courtroom carrying it,"

Christine says. "But when I opened it up, there'd be a breast pump, bottles, nursing pads, and all that. Kind of blew the professional image."

Packing Your Breastfeeding Kit

- Supplies for expressing milk can be brought to work in a briefcase, tote bag, lunch box, brown bag, insulated bag, or the cooler you are using for storage, and can contain:
- Containers for milk storage (plastic or glass jars, bottles, disposable bottles and bags, plastic bags with ties).
- Breast shields or pads.
- Breast pump (if used).
- Plastic breast shield to collect milk leaking from other breast while expressing.
- Soap or disposable hand wipes (or a damp washcloth stored in a plastic bag).
- Towels (paper or cloth) to place on your lap.
- Self-adhesive tags or adhesive tape for labeling and dating milk.
- Blue ice in a cooler (if you don't have an available refrigerator).

Hint: Keep extras in your desk or locker—pads, washcloths, shields, containers (make sure they are tightly covered to keep them clean or sterile, or use disposable nurser bag). Also, keep a sweater at work in case you need a quick coverup for an unscheduled leak.

Bottles and Supplements

Many mothers decide not to try to supply 100 percent breastmilk while they are at work and instead provide formula for missed feedings. How well your body adjusts to this routine and how much your milk supply is affected will depend on the age of your child, how well your milk supply has stabilized, and making sure you breastfeed frequently when at home. Many women are able to establish this routine quite comfortably.

Jane L. provided formula for both morning and afternoon feedings; however, she breastfed her baby at noon.

"It makes it much easier on me. I have enough things I get upset about, and I decided I'm not going to get upset about breastfeeding. It's not going to kill her if she takes formula once in a while. I'm happy with whatever she does. Even when she decides she doesn't want me anymore, it's been a wonderful experience and I'm not going to feel bad. Having a baby and breastfeeding is wonderful, and you have to do whatever works for you."

"If an emergency arose, I didn't feel so strongly that my child could not have a drop of formula," says Alice K. "I didn't feel like he was going to die if he had formula because I had to get back to work."

"If you want to nurse your baby and pump and give only breastmilk, you can do that," said Elizabeth C., a pediatric nurse who breastfed two babies and also counsels breastfeeding women. "If you want to nurse during the hours you're at home and leave a bottle of formula when you're gone, the baby will nutritionally do fine, and your body should adjust to that kind of situation. I know lots of mothers who nurse morning, evening, and night and leave formula for during the day. You need to do what you're most comfortable doing, not what your husband or mother or baby-sitter wants you to do.

"If you're trying to nurse on a full-time basis and work full-time because that's what someone else wants you to do, it's not going to be a pleasurable experience. The key is to enjoy your baby. When it becomes a chore for you, it's no longer fun, and your baby suffers in the long run."

If your baby will be given a bottle while you are at work, you don't want to spring this change on her. Most mothers introduce practice bottles before returning to work, so the baby can get used to sucking on a different nipple. In a 1984 survey conducted at the University of Wisconsin-Milwaukee (Maclaughlin and Strelnick), mothers offered bottles as early as one week and as late as twenty-four weeks, with six weeks being the average age for starting the baby on the bottle. Breastmilk was used by about half of the mothers; the others used water or formula. The mothers who were planning to use breastmilk in the workday bottles did not omit any feedings and introduced a bottle of breastmilk. The women who planned to use formula omitted breastfeedings to make sure the baby would accept a formula substitute when the time came.

"I started using my pump maybe a little too early, when she was about two weeks. But at first I used it to express some milk if I was really engorged, or to get a little supply of milk in the freezer so if I wanted to get away or go out I could leave her with a sitter or with my husband. One time I went to the grocery store and thought that she was fine, but she cried the whole time I was gone. So I had left my husband in a bad situation. After that I started expressing milk because I thought, No way I'm going to leave him like that—it was a desperate feeling for him."

Finding a bottle-feeding system your baby likes may take a little trial and error. There are numerous glass, plastic, and disposable options, and this choice may depend in part on whether you are using the bottles for breastmilk storage as well. Plastic is considered best for storage, since some of the milk components tend to stick to glass. And though disposable bags are handy for storage, they can develop small holes when frozen.

Rubber nipples can be confusing to infants at first, because no matter how closely they claim to replicate mother's, the suckling action is different. The material (whether rubber, latex, or silicone) is less flexible: the flow may be more rapid; or the holes may be too small. If the flow is too rapid, causing the baby to sputter or choke, you'll have to discard the nipple. If the hole is too small (the baby seems frustrated or takes much longer to feed than when she is at the breast), enlarge it by heating a needle over a flame and passing it through the opening.

The Nuk nipple claims to be designed most like the human breast. Ultimately, though, your baby will probably make the final decision, and you may have to experiment a bit.

"At first it was hard for her to take a bottle—she didn't want to. I tried every kind of nipple on the market, and what I found she liked the best was Pur. It's not the Nuk formation; it's just a regular standard nipple, made of clear plastic, and it's really a lot softer than the brown rubber nipples. In fact, I sucked on it myself to see how much softer it was."

Some mothers give a daily bottle in preparation for their return to work. Or you can arrange a bottle-feeding during a time when you plan to be out of the house anyway, on an errand or at a social activity. It is a good idea, at least some of the time, for the bottle to be offered by your spouse, mother, babysitter, or ideally, the same caregiver who will be taking care of your baby while you are at work. (In fact, some breastfed babies won't take a bottle from Mom—it's breast or nothing.) Some parents leave their baby with the workday caregiver for a trial run or two in advance of the real thing. This can help to make the actual transition more comfortable for both you and your baby.

"My husband is so delighted about this baby, and he wants so much to be a part of it," says Brenda N. "It was such a neat time feeding her; her expressions and her smiles and things were so much fun. I felt like I was the lucky one, getting to enjoy all that, and I wanted him to be able to feed her. He feeds her once every three or fours day. And it got her used to taking a bottle.

"As soon as I got some milk expressed, I got my husband to start trying to give her the bottle. The first time she really threw a fit for him, but she'd take it from me. Then the next time we tried he got her to take the bottle and that was really a mark in history for us, because he wanted so badly to do this. She was about two and a half weeks old."

As to formula, give yourself time to experiment in case your baby is allergic or does not tolerate a particular type.

Each infant formula claims to have a nutritional composition that is closest to mother's milk. Basically, all formulas are made with a soy base or with a cow's milk base. Most babies do fine with a cow's milk formula, although there are some physicians who prefer to avoid cow's milk derivatives because of their implication in allergies. You will want to consult with your pediatrician to help with your decision and to evaluate your baby's response to the formula you choose.

Formulas come in powder, concentrated liquid, and ready-to-feed forms. The ready-to-feed form is obviously the most convenient, but the powder form is the most economical, because it can be made up one feeding at a time and there is no waste. Also, the powder preparations have a longer shelf life, and it has been suggested that powders are better tolerated by the infant because more heat is used in their manufacture.

However, when you're working and breastfeeding, your time is also a precious commodity. Said one mother: "At first I wanted to be real economical, so we used the powder. I wanted to do it all right, trying to be the perfect mom. So I'd boil the water and wait for it to cool and then mix the powder and I always made a mess, and it took a lot of time. After a while I finally decided that my time was worth something, so we started buying the premade stuff in cans."

Tips on Infant Formula

1. *Check the expiration date* on the container (indicated as "use by" or "use before"). Do not buy or feed formula beyond the expiration date. If you accidentally buy formula that is out-of-date at the time of purchase, return it to the store for exchange or refund.

2. *Sterilize equipment and water* used to prepare formula, unless your pediatrician or health professional says it is not necessary.

3. Formula is available in *three forms:* ready-to-feed, concentrated liquid, or powder. The concentrated liquid

and powder must be mixed with water according to the instructions on the container.

4. *Do not refrigerate or reheat* a bottle once the baby has nursed from it. Discard any unused portions of formula.

5. An opened can of liquid formula can be *stored safely in the refrigerator for up to forty-eight hours* (if transferred to a glass container, tightly covered and refrigerated immediately). Formula that has been prepared from concentrate or powder should be refrigerated and used within twenty-four hours.

6. *Do not freeze* formula.

NURSING PADS: DON'T LEAVE HOME WITHOUT 'EM

"I'll never forget the time I was talking to my male boss and my milk let down. I could feel the wet spot spreading out on my blouse. Luckily I had a legal pad in my hand, so I quickly covered myself with it."

Keep nursing pads in your desk drawer, purse, and briefcase. You can buy boxes of disposable pads in most drugstores and maternity shops. However, if you leak often or heavily, you might find that disposables retain the moisture and cause skin irritation. Washable pads, which are usually sold in boxes of six, may keep you drier because the cotton draws the moisture away from the skin—and they are reusable. Buy a few of each type to see which you prefer.

Nursing pads are contour-shaped or flat with a cut area that allows you to mold them to your own contour. Again, experimentation is the best way to decide which works best. An alternative to breast pads is using cut pieces of a mini sanitary pad. The sticky tape on the underside clings nicely to the bra. Be aware that breast pads show through some white blouses and light or sheer fabrics, necessitating a slip or camisole.

BREAST CUPS AND SHIELDS

As mentioned in Chapter Two, breast shields can also be used to catch milk that leaks from one breast while the other is nursing or being pumped. If you do tend to leak while you pump or express, a shield may be essential to protect your work clothing. Discard any milk that leaks into the shield and wash the shield thoroughly because bacteria grows easily in the warm environment.

Because plastic shields reduce the flow of air to the breast, it is not a good idea to wear them all the time. Many mothers use them only when they are nursing or pumping and at times in their jobs when they don't want to take any chances. For example, for her monthly financial reports to her company's board of directors, Gretchen T. wears plastic shields during the hour or two she is in the meeting and picks that day to wear a suit or a blouse and cardigan.

To Prevent Those Untimely Wet Spots . . .

- Wear milk cups
- Change breast pads right before a meeting or special event
- Wear a sweater or jacket

Dressing for Success Breastfeeding-Wise

"If I wore a blouse and skirt it was easier. There were a couple of dresses I wore that I had to take off completely. But since I could lock my office, it was okay. Once I got over being a little embarrassed, even though I was by myself, it just really didn't matter; it was really easy."

What you wear to work won't matter so much if you have a private, lockable office or room in which to pump. But most women find they need clothing that facilitates pumping and provides a measure of discretion when there are other people around. Blouses or dresses that open in the front have an obvious advantage, although when using a pump some women like to slip the pump up under a sweater or shirt. Nursing slips, available in maternity shops, have a detachable flap that lets down to expose the breast. You can also wear a camisole.

The latest in nursing attire are blouses or shirts with zippers that run the full length of the garment on each side over the breast area. The zippers are attractively stitched to look like part of the blouse's styling or are concealed under pleats. Other tops have side openings that are practically invisible.

Everyone leaks at one time or another. When choosing clothing, consider patterns or plaids, which camouflage wet spots better than solid colors do.

Frankly, clothing for working/breastfeeding women is not the hottest fashion trend. It may be difficult to find tops or dresses that suit your tastes and breastfeeding needs. The best places to look for nursing blouses and shirts are maternity shops, but don't count on finding a wide selection even there. There are also patterns available. (You've got to be kidding! Spare time to sew?) In addition, a number of mail-order businesses, many of them mother-owned cottage industries, now offer selections of attractive tops and dresses for breastfeeding women.

Most women are anxious to return to their regular wardrobes as soon as possible. You probably have plenty of clothes suitable for nursing and pumping at work. With these, plus a few new items bought with your breastfeeding needs in mind, you'll probably get by without having to spend a lot of money on specialty designs.

5

Back to Work— Your Plan

"You really have to be dedicated to working and breastfeeding. You have to believe in what you're doing. If you're doing it just because everybody else said you should, it will be real hard."

"It helps to have supportive people around you. There were times when I'd get discouraged, and I was fortunate to have people around me who told me to hang in there."

"You need to relax and enjoy it. I'm afraid I didn't do that as much as I hope to be able to the next time. I was so tense about it—'Will I be able to pump enough?' 'What if he needs another bottle that I don't have?' "

"I talked to enough people and got up my confidence and decided that it was going to work. Once

*I decided it was right, I could do anything—I bet
that was ninety percent of making it successful."*

*"If you really want to do it, you can do it. But I
don't think you should totally commit yourself if
the time is not right or there are circumstances
that make you unable to do it. And you shouldn't
stress yourself out if you can't. Definitely try it,
but don't worry about it and don't feel guilty if it
doesn't work out."*

*"The biggest problem is people who can't under-
stand why you're going to all this trouble."*

*"I felt like I was being pulled in two directions—
my baby tugging on one arm and my job on the
other. After a while I realized that it was* me *who
was doing most of the pulling."*

When should you go back to work? This is a big question,
and for breastfeeding mothers, a very important one. If the standard six-week maternity leave is sealed in cement, you may
have no choice. Or you may have the option of extending your
leave, either with or without the guarantee that the same job
will be waiting for you when you return. Perhaps a promotion
is in the offing, to be gobbled up by someone else if you're not
around. Maybe you can't afford to give up your salary. Or, as
with many women, you may simply want to get back to your
job.

Situations like this place new mothers under increased
pressure to return to work as soon as possible. You feel torn—
you would like to be at home a little longer with your baby, but
the workplace beckons. It is most important that you don't
spend the time you do have worrying about what will happen
when it's over. Going back to work does not mean that your
wonderful relationship with your baby is over. Rather, a new

phase of your parenting is beginning, and for many women, one that is every bit as rewarding as the first.

Many women say breastfeeding gives them a special link and an instant closeness with their babies that helps to compensate for the hours during which they are apart. And by pumping and saving breastmilk at work, they are meeting their babies' needs during the times they cannot provide for them in person. For these women, the rewards outweigh the inconvenience and extra hassle. But no one says it's easy—or that it's for everyone.

Beware of the supermother. You know her? She's the part of you that hangs over your shoulder and reminds you of everything you "should" be doing. She usually expects too much, devises incredibly impossible rules, and makes you feel terrible if you don't live up to them. If she is the one who's telling you to work and breastfeed, you may be setting yourself up for a lot of unnecessary frustration and guilt. Working and breastfeeding is tricky enough for you to handle without this relentless ideal lurking in the background. How you time your return to work, and the particular working/breastfeeding pattern you devise, will be of your own making—self-styled according to how, when, and where you work, the particular environment in which you do so, and the distance you travel to your job.

The most outstanding characteristic of the women we interviewed who balance working and breastfeeding in a way that gives them pleasure and satisfaction is that they are relaxed. Wait a minute, you protest. You mean on top of everything else I have to be laid back, too?

No, but you do need to ease up on yourself and avoid making excessive demands or setting rigid expectations. The women we spoke with were busy. They made no bones about the difficulty of orchestrating days and evenings so that every minute counts. Their schedules are tight—but they are not. They are less frenetic than they are tenacious. They know that exhaustion will sabotage breastfeeding. They have learned, often the hard way, how to change course as well as the importance of staying flexible. And long ago they gave up the idea of being supermoms. They have no qualms about relying on lots of support from family, friends, and coworkers. They don't feel an ounce of guilt about hiring someone to clean the house and do the laundry.

TIMING

There are advantages to waiting several months before you go back to work. By then you will probably have regained all of your prebirth get-up-and-go, you will be getting a decent night's sleep, your milk supply will be well established, and most of the problems encountered in the early days of breast-feeding will be behind you. Much of the weight you gained during pregnancy will be gone, so you won't need to buy a new wardrobe (even though you'd probably like to). Also, at four months your baby is likely to be down to four or five feedings a day. This means you may have to pump or make arrangements to nurse only once during the workday—clearly more convenient than the two to three pumpings necessary to work and to breastfeed a six-week-old infant.

However, waiting this long seems to be a luxury the majority of working/breastfeeding women cannot afford. In a survey conducted at the University of Nebraska Medical Center (Auerbach and Guss, 1984), over six-hundred-fifty women from forty-nine states and five foreign countries reported having worked and breastfed. Of those women, 76 percent were back on the job before the baby was thirteen weeks old, with the most common age being ten weeks. Mothers who returned to work before their babies were sixteen weeks old weaned them earlier than mothers who returned between sixteen weeks and four months.

According to the Nebraska study, the specific occupation was not significantly related to how well working and breast-feeding progressed. The biggest issues were the timing of return and the number of hours worked. Part-time workers tended to breastfeed longer than women who were on a full-time (forty hours or more) schedule. However, *when* these mothers returned to work had a greater effect on how long the baby breastfed than did the number of daily work hours. Mothers who returned to work full time before the infant was sixteen weeks weaned their babies before the first year. Full-time working mothers who waited until the baby was at least four months nursed longer than part-time working mothers who returned to work before sixteen weeks.

These statistics are not intended as predictions of how successful your working/breastfeeding experience will be. Nor should you feel you won't be successful if you return to work when your baby is six weeks old. But it helps to know that the demands you face have been shared by many other women with varying results. Many of the women surveyed said that they "cherished the nursing relationship," but also noted that they had to work hard to continue. Many reported that working had a negative effect on breastfeeding, but none said that breastfeeding exerted a negative effect on their jobs.

Supermother you do not have to be. Determined, yes. Imaginative, definitely. But most of all, you've got to be flexible. Begin with the best plan you can devise—knowing that your relaxed attitude will be the fulcrum that keeps all the pieces in balance.

"A lot of people I talk to really get spooked, and I don't know why," says Leslie F., a full-time office manager who worked and breastfed until her daughter was six months old. "Some women worry so much that it affects their supply. To me, it's just such a neat thing and so natural—something that I can provide, something that my baby needs. Maybe if I had nursed her longer it might have been better, but hey!—I gave Ivy the best I had to offer at the time."

THINKING IT THROUGH

The first steps in your planning process are to: 1. Evaluate yourself and your job; 2. Evaluate your work environment; 3. Find good, supportive child care.

Evaluate Yourself and Your Job

1. How do you feel about your job? Do you want to continue with this job or do you wish you had another one?
2. If you are dissatisfied with your job, is a change possible (either a move within your current company or a new job)? If not, develop a list of your concerns and constructive suggestions for improvement, and present these to your employer. Arrange a meeting with your employer either before or during your maternity leave. At that time, discuss your plans for working and breastfeeding and your ideas for improving your job situation.
3. Do you feel guilty about going back to work? You're not alone. Many women share these feelings, along with anxiety about being separated from their infants. Find and talk with other working mothers. There is no reason to feel guilty about wanting to have a job. The better you feel about yourself, the better parent you will be.
4. Do you have a choice about when to return to work? Financially, can you afford to wait a few months? Make a list of your expenses, income, and savings.
5. Can you work part time for a month or two until your baby begins to take fewer feedings each day? Discuss this possibility with your employer, and be sure to ask what effect part time hours will have on your company's benefit programs. If you are in school, consider reducing your class hours for one term.
6. Can you work flex-time? Or can you split shifts with someone else, or work out an arrangement for trading hours? If possible, discuss this with your co-workers and supervisor before your maternity leave begins.

7. Can you bring your baby to work with you? Before you discuss this with your employer, work out a written plan describing exactly how and where you will care for the baby, and how you will handle special situations (see Chapter Six).

8. Can you work at home until your baby is older? Again, it is a good idea to have a written plan when you discuss this option with your employer.

9. Do you enjoy breastfeeding? Are you proud and happy with this method of feeding your baby? Are you comfortable telling people you breastfeed? Are you able to express your milk manually, and will you be comfortable pumping at your workplace? Are you anxious for breastfeeding to continue?

10. Are you and your baby healthy? Is your milk supply well established? Will your baby accept a bottle of either formula or your breastmilk?

[Renee A., a registered nurse and education director, worked and nursed her daughter for twenty-two months. Because she shared an office with an agreeable coworker, Renee was able to bring Holly with her to work for the first five months.]

"Normally our office doors were not closed, so when I brought Holly we talked about the door being closed so she would not disturb the clients. But it was understood that anyone could come in—it was still 'open-door' policy. I had a couch in my office, and that made it really handy. That was where she took her naps, and when she was awake I could prop her up. I brought toys in and kept a bag of toys at the office.

"I started going back to work a little bit when she was two weeks old, for an occasional meeting, and I took her with me. Then I went back full time at six weeks. She went to board meetings, and the board understood that it was real important for me to have her with me. I breastfed all the time. Holly ate through all of our staff meetings. I felt very comfortable—it was an all-female staff, and our whole purpose is women's health care, so it was a real supportive system."

"If you really believe in it, you're going to be able to do it. I think people get lots of messages that it's 'not professional' or 'demeaning,' but you have to know that what you're doing is very important."

"It made me sit down and spend some time with my baby. If I had bottle-fed her, I know that at five-thirty in the evening, when everybody came home and I was trying to do dinner and my two-and-a-half-year-old was wanting to tell me everything that happened during the day, it would have been real easy to put the baby on the couch with a bottle propped up. When you breastfeed, you have to sit down, put your feet up; you're oblivious to the dust on the coffee table and you spend some real one-on-one time. A real special quiet time."

"On my first day back at work, one of my coworkers said, 'It must be hard to leave your baby like this.' My response was that staying home was much harder than being at work. I was glad to be back, although I did miss my little boy."

Evaluate Your Work Environment

Use these questions and comments to examine how well your job situation will accommodate breastfeeding, and to form the basis for your discussion of your working/breast-feeding routine with your employer.

1. What are your work and travel hours?

   Travel time to work_____
   Travel time to child's caregiver_____
   Hours spent at work_____

   TOTAL HOURS AWAY FROM HOME_____

If your total exceeds eight hours and you return to work when your baby is less than twelve weeks old, you will need to pump or nurse two to three times during your workday.

2. How is your lunch break structured?

Is it flexible or at a specific time?
How long is your break?
Can you leave your work area?
Can you leave the premises?
Can you pack a lunch?
Can you get a sitter near work so you can lunch there?

3. How are your work breaks structured?

Are they flexible or specified?
How long are they?
Can you leave the work area?

For two to three pumpings per day, you will need two breaks of fifteen to twenty minutes, and at least thirty minutes for lunch (if your lunch break is this short, you will probably need to bring your lunch from home). You can manage your pumping schedule around specified times, but it is much easier when the breaks are flexible. Discuss a flexible break time with your supervisor, or find a coworker who is willing to swap with you now and then (for example, when you let down unexpectedly and have another half hour to go before break).

You will need to leave the work area and find a quiet, private spot to express your milk.

If your child-care provider lives close by, you can nurse on your lunch break.

If your child-care provider is willing to bring the baby to you, you can nurse at lunch in the car or in a private spot in the workplace.

4. What are your duties?

> Are your duties tightly structured or planned?
> Is your job high pressured?
> Do you have deadlines to meet?
> Is your routine often interrupted?
> Do you have meetings to attend?
> Are meetings ever before or after hours?
> Do you have lunch meetings?

> List any circumstances that might interfere with a regular, daily routine. Even if your schedule is absolutely unpredictable, you can manage working and breastfeeding as long as you can slip off two to three times a day for fifteen to twenty minutes. Could you go out to your nearby car to pump? In Chapter Six we will discuss specific strategies in more detail.

5. What do you wear to work?

> Can you wear clothing that facilitates pumping and breastfeeding?
> If you wear a uniform, is it designed to allow access to your breasts?
> If not, can you alter the uniform? Can you wear another style?

6. What is the physical setting of your workplace?

> Is there a refrigerator you can use?
> Can you carry your own cooler for storage?
> Is there a private place for you to pump?
> Are the rest rooms private?
> Are the rest rooms clean?
> Can you borrow someone's office?

> Is there a spot near your workplace where you can go to pump? As a breastfeeding mother, you deserve a place that is both comfortable and clean. You should

not have to "sneak off" or settle for marginal conditions in order to provide your baby's food. Frankness and confidence when communicating your needs to your employer should bring results if you are having trouble locating a spot in which to pump. Virtually all buildings have someplace where a person can go to be alone. If you are meeting resistance in your efforts to set up a working/breastfeeding routine, you might try taking your concerns to the personnel department or going through employee grievance channels if there are any. Also, see Chapter Eleven for legal alternatives that may be open to you.

7. What are the attitudes of your supervisor and coworkers toward breastfeeding?

Do other women coworkers breastfeed?
Does your employer have children?
Were they or are they breastfed?
What is your employer's reaction to your plan?
Does your company have a high regard for the family?
Can you leave for family emergencies?
Will your union support you?
What is your company policy?

Before you meet with your supervisor to present your breastfeeding plans, make sure you have a clear idea of what you want to accomplish, how you plan to do it, and what specific problems you anticipate for which you would like his/her assistance. Prepare notes in advance, and bring these notes with you. If you cannot gain the backing of your supervisor, take your requests to the personnel department.

8. Do you have the support of family and friends?

Is your spouse enthusiastic about your working and breastfeeding?

Is he informed about breastfeeding?
Is he available to drive the baby to the care provider?
Would he bring the baby to you at lunch?
Does he share in the household duties?
Do you have other working/breastfeeding friends?

The best sources of encouragement and approval will be other working/breastfeeding mothers. Form a loose organization or a formal one. Go to lunch together regularly (or, rather, grab a quick bite after you pump). Have dinner once a month (this is difficult but fun if you can pull it off). Telephone each other; create your own hot line. Talk and listen.

FINDING CHILD CARE

The knowledge that your baby is in good hands is the key to your transition back to work. Add to that a caregiver who is supportive of your breastfeeding, and you have the makings of many good days. To find the right person(s) to care for your baby, start early. Begin looking at least three months before you plan to return to work—earlier if you are starting from scratch with no leads. It takes time to call friends, your child care resource and referral agency, follow up on their suggestions, place ads in the newspaper, conduct interviews.

You may not make the right child care choice the first time out. Be willing to change care providers if you're dissatisfied, or if something simply "doesn't feel right." Also, keep in mind that the caregiver you choose when your child is an infant may not be the best person for your child as she grows older. When she begins to play and interact with other children, you will want to take a second look at the child care setting to make sure the environment is stimulating and diverse enough for an older, active toddler.

There are three basic types of child care: a caregiver who comes to your home (in-home care), a family child care home, and a child care center. Your decision will depend on the kind of care that is available to you, how you personally feel about the people and the child care environment, and how they respond to your baby. Since you will be asking your care provider to help you by adjusting the baby's feedings to your breastfeeding schedule, "holding the baby off" if you are late, storing and managing your breastmilk, and perhaps bringing the baby to you for a feeding, you will want to find someone who shares your commitment to breastfeeding.

Caregivers in your home. When someone comes to your home, you have the advantage of one-on-one care, no transport or packing supplies, and less pressure in the morning to get the baby dressed and ready to go. However, you must find someone you trust implicitly. This caregiver will be alone in your home, with no other adults (or children) to monitor her activities. Choose an in-home caregiver very carefully, relying on several references and, if possible, the recommendation of people you know personally. It is a good idea to arrange a backup, too, for times when your regular caregiver is sick or out of town.

Child care homes. Typically these are situations in which a mother of young children or an older mother cares for a limited number of children in her own home. If she is licensed by the city or state, there will be a limit on the number of children she can take. Here, your child should receive individualized attention in an atmosphere much like your own home. It is important to ask how many children are full time, how many are part time, and how many are "drop-ins" (brought to the home occasionally). Find out what types of activities the children participate in and if they are ever taken on outings. Ask if the care provider belongs to any type of community child care network, association, child care database, or is on the Child Care Food Programs. This information tells you whether she is sponsored, supervised, has backup if she is ill or on vacation, and has a source for new materials and supportive services such as in-service training and help with problems.

Child care centers. There are usually a lot of children in child care centers, but the good centers have enough adults to go around. Infants should be in small groups, in a separate room, with their own primary caregiver. The kind of care your baby receives will depend on how many babies each caregiver is responsible for and the quality of care she offers. Child care centers offer advantages to older children because the day is often structured around a variety of activities, many educational, and the environment is like a nursery school. The biggest problem with large child care centers is that they are germ and virus bonanzas—contagious diseases come with the territory when little children are around, and in child care centers illness can run rampant. However, a well-equipped, loving child care center can be a wonderful find. As your baby gets older, this kind of facility will be able to meet her growing needs for play, enrichment activities and materials, and friendships with a variety of children.

Licensed or Unlicensed?

Many states have particular standards governing child care facilities, insurance, qualifications of providers, and the ages and number of children. To find your local, city, or state licensing agency, contact your department of health. However, a license is not a guarantee that a particular center or home will deliver the care you want. Ultimately, the decision is yours.

Finding Child Care Providers

Begin by contacting one of the following (depending on where you live): your city, county, or state department of health, human resources, social services, or children and family services; local child care information or referral services; local junior league; your church; friends; coworkers with children; relatives. Place a notice on the bulletin board at your workplace, your church, neighborhood grocery or children's stores. Place an advertisement in the newspaper.

Note: When you place a notice or ad, give your phone number and first name only. When respondents call, ask for their references first. Tell them you will call back after you have checked the references, and then call each reference. This will weed out those who are not really interested and also save you the trouble of interviewing anyone whose references are unsatisfactory. Conduct initial interviews by phone, meeting candidates in person when you have narrowed down your choices. If you can afford an automatic phone answering machine, you can save a lot of time by having respondents introduce themselves and list their references on the tape.

Sample Advertisements—Classified Section of Newspaper

Child care needed for a six-week-old girl in your loving home on the north side near Eighth and Main. Monday–Friday, 7:30 A.M.–5:30 P.M. Call Jane after 5:30 at 326-1111.

Child Care needed in my home or yours for twelve-week-old baby boy in the Springdale area. Monday–Wednesday, 7:00 A.M.–6:00 P.M. Call Debra after 6:00 at 377-4780.

Visit the Child Care Provider

It might be easier to schedule your first appointment after hours, when the care provider is not busy with her charges. This will give you a chance to ask general questions, read through any written material about the center or home, and talk with the provider about your baby. You can then go back later to observe the children and to see how she responds to them. Bring your baby with you on this visit. After your baby is enrolled, you should have unlimited access to him or her. It is a legal right.

What follows are questions you should ask the care provider and questions you should ask yourself as you talk with her and look around. This list has been consolidated from a number of sources.

What to Ask About Child Care

1. *General information.* Will you accept my child? Is there an opening? What are the hours? What are the costs? How many children are cared for there (and are they full time or part time)? What is the ratio of adults to children? Is there an adult present at all times? How long has the center or home been in operation? If an individual, how long have you been caring for children? What qualifications, training, and experience do you (and the other caregivers) have? Are you licensed? Are you a member of a community child care network? Do you have written materials I can read? Can you provide three references? Do you or any of the care providers smoke on the premises? What is your policy on illness?

2. *Questions about child care.* (Not all of these questions will apply to your particular situation.) Do you have children? Did you breastfeed? Are you able to bring the child to me at work? Will you call me at work when the baby needs to be fed? If I am late, can you try to hold off the baby's feeding until I get there to nurse her? How do you feel about using my frozen or refrigerated breastmilk for feedings?

3. *Situational questions.* What if my child is sick? If another woman came to your door and said I had told her to pick up Eric, what would you do? How do you handle times when the baby cries all day? Do you think babies are "spoiled" by being held too much? How do you give the baby her bottle? How much time will my child spend in the crib? What will you do with her when she's not in the crib? Do you take the children outdoors? For child care homes: What do you do with the other children if one gets hurt and needs medical attention? What happens if you get sick?

4. *Questions to ask yourself.* When you and your baby visit her, how does the caregiver respond to her? Does

she greet your baby in a warm, loving way? How do you feel when she is holding your child? Can you form a partnership with this person? Will you be able to communicate with her and express your feelings and concerns directly, unapologetically? Is she interested in your baby and your experiences? Is she open to all your questions? When you talk about your baby, does she ask questions in return? Does she want to know about you? Will she be supportive of your special needs as a working/breastfeeding mother? Does she seem to think what you are doing is great, or does it sound like "a lot of trouble" to her?

5. *Physical setting.* Do the children seem content and happy? Is the environment clean and safe (it *will* be messy, because kids stay there)? Where are the cribs located (in a quiet spot)? Are the cribs clean and free of toys and pillows? Is the home child-proofed (outlets covered, poisons locked in cabinets, no sharp objects, toys in good repair)? Do the furnishings and large toys look stable and nonhazardous? Is the temperature comfortable? Are there first-aid supplies and emergency phone numbers handy? Does the home have smoke detectors (including those mounted above stairways and over doors of rooms where children sleep)? Does the caregiver know how to resuscitate a choking or nonbreathing infant?

6. When all the questions are said and done, stand back and take a deep breath. Now, ask yourself: How do *you* feel about this care for your baby? Is this the right place or the wrong one? Listen carefully to your instincts—they're the best guidepost of all.

Once you have hired a caregiver, don't expect everything to be perfect, or if it is, that this will last forever. Things can change. Drop by unannounced from time to time just to check.

HOUSEKEEPING SERVICE CAN BE A LIFESAVER

This is not the time to be a housework heroine. If you can afford to spend a bit of your salary on an extra pair of hands, it will be worth every penny. You may decide to hire someone for a few hours a week to vacuum and clean the bathroom and scrape the crust off the kitchen. Or you might be able to afford the luxury of having a person come every day to straighten up, do laundry, start dinner. Any help you can get will take the edge off (not to mention the dust), and give you some well-deserved time to lazily nurse your baby.

Tips on Hiring a Housekeeper

- Word-of-mouth is usually a very reliable source.
- Place an ad in the classified section of the newspaper.
- Check the classified ads under "Employment Wanted."
- Contact your local high school or college job-placement center.
- Contact an established cleaning service. These people are usually bonded (check the policy for expiration date and amount of coverage).
- Ask for three references, and call them all before you interview the candidate. Ask references: Is this person thorough? How does s/he respond when you make corrections or ask that a particular job be done? Does s/he have a key to your home? Does s/he come to work on the days promised?
- Find out what the housekeeper charges and compare this fee with what friends and coworkers pay for similar services.
- If your housekeeper works for a cleaning service, you do not have to withhold taxes or pay social security. If the person works independently and will be paid more than fifty dollars each quarter, you need to pay social

security and file annual W-2 forms for that employee. To find out how to do this, call the federal tax information number (toll free) listed in your phone directory under "U.S. Government Offices."

- Decide how many hours you think it will take to clean your home and hire the housekeeper for that period. If the housekeeper charges a flat fee, ask how long s/he expects to take. Whatever your fee basis is, you will judge on how well the job is done, anyway.
- Be specific about what you want done. Make a list.
- Keep a notepad handy to jot down jobs you would like done the next time. Ask the housekeeper to check the notepad each time. The housekeeper can then use the notepad for messages and problems and to tell you about supplies you need, etc.
- If your housekeeper will be responsible for shopping, leave detailed lists and money and ask for receipts.
- You can establish a good relationship with a housekeeper if you regard him or her as a professional employed by you to perform a valuable job, *not* as someone on whom you are foisting your dirty work. This attitude will also help you to communicate as employer to employee and make management and problem-solving less awkward. As time goes by, remember to give raises in salary and paid vacation days.

BACK TO WORK (ALMOST) — A "TRIAL RUN"

About two weeks before she returned to her full-time office job, Ruth E. gave four-week-old Amy a bottle of breastmilk once or twice a day. The baby accepted the bottle easily. "I also started her on a little bit of formula, to see how she would react in case I needed it for backup," Ruth says. "I was really surprised—she didn't show any preference between bottle and breast.

"The week before I went back to work, I took her to

the baby-sitter on Tuesday and Wednesday for half days, and Thursday and Friday for full days, just to get her used to it. But it was more for my sake—to find out if the milk I was expressing was enough and to see how much formula I needed to bring. I expressed milk while she was at the sitter, just like I would do if I were back at work. Those days were pretty good indicators, except that when I was at home I got more milk than when I went back to work. At home I had more time to express milk, I was a little bit more relaxed about it, and I didn't have to worry about confining myself to a certain time of day."

Introducing practice bottles a week or two before you return to work will help your baby acclimate to the change and also assure you that your baby will, in fact, get nourishment while you are away. Some mothers introduce a bottle of breastmilk in place of a feeding; others combine breast and bottle in one feeding. In either case, be sure you express or pump your breasts completely.

When the bottle is offered by another person (father, grandparent, caregiver), the baby gets accustomed to being fed by others. In the meantime, you are pumping and saving, just as you will do at work.

Let's say your baby is older (over four months) when you return to work and you are planning to provide formula for the missed feeding without expressing milk at work. You may want to begin omitting breastfeedings at the same time of day your baby will receive formula. This will alter your own production of breastmilk and assist your body in establishing a new routine. This will also give you time to observe how your baby tolerates the formula. However, to omit feedings without pumping and still maintain an adequate supply of milk for all the other feedings, you must have a very well-established milk supply.

If time permits, schedule several half-day "practice runs" with your baby's caregiver, including feedings and naps. And when you return to work full time, consider doing so on Friday or midweek if you can. A shorter first week will help make the transition easier, and you'll have the weekend to recover.

A Simulated Work Day

- Get up about forty-five minutes earlier than usual.
- Breastfeed (don't rush).
- Eat a good breakfast.
- Dress your baby and you (in that order).
- Pack baby's bag (or pack it the night before).
- Pack your own supplies (briefcase, breastfeeding kit, lunch).
- Travel to the caregiver (or plan to have her come to your home).
- Allow enough time to talk with caregiver and give any special instructions.
- You may want to plan time to nurse baby there.
- Travel to your workplace.

How are you doing so far? Did you arrive at work in reasonably good shape (hair combed, two matching shoes, breathing normally)? If not, you will need to allow more time, or do more preparation the evening before. As time goes by, you will be able to streamline your exit and catch a little extra shut-eye.

- Express milk during your simulated day just as you would at work.
- If possible, spend as much of the day outside the home as you can.
- If your work breaks are not flexible, try to stick to that schedule.
- If your work breaks are flexible, note the times that are best for expression.
- Save and store your breastmilk.
- Note times when you become engorged, and when you leak.
- Don't forget to eat a nourishing lunch.

- Return to the caregiver at the time you will ordinarily pick up your baby.
- Breastfeed right away if possible, or as soon as you arrive home.

Is your baby ready to eat? If not, is it because the caregiver fed her too close to your arrival? Suggest that the caregiver offer a pacifier, a little warm water, or an ounce or two of milk to tide the baby over until you arrive.

How did the caregiver's day go? How many feedings did your baby take? Was there enough milk or formula? Did your baby accept the bottle well? Does the caregiver have any questions about thawing or warming your breastmilk? How many diapers did she use? What supplies did you forget to pack?

Does your baby seem content and cared for? (Remember, she may be upset at first if she is very hungry.) Count the diapers left—was your baby changed often enough? Is the diaper area clean? Does your baby sleep well at night (or is she awake because she slept all day)? Is she clean when you pick her up?

Packing Baby's Bag

- Diapers: pack two more than you ordinarily use in a day
- Two changes of clothes
- Plastic bags for dirty clothes or diapers
- Formula (amount will depend on whether it is used for feedings or for backup only)
- Pacifier
- Baby wipes
- Extra empty bottle (clean or sterilized)
- Toys
- Your breastmilk, frozen or refrigerated (put this in just before you leave)

Congratulations! You're on final countdown.

6

Under Way

"The hardest thing about breastfeeding is needing to be there and the number of hours in the day it requires. But it's such a short period in your life."

"First and foremost is to get the support of your employer. If you're agitated about what you're trying to do, that's a major problem. And you need to be flexible—that's really a key. If you're so rigid that you can't flex around the baby's time, or the baby can't flex a little around you, then you've got a problem. If you're trying to nurse a baby and you're needed at your job, that's a stressful situation for all concerned."

"Pumping and saving milk works fine for lots of women. If you are pumping at work you need privacy and the time to feel comfortable about what you're doing, and not just rushed, rushed, rushed all the time."

"I knew a lawyer who had to express in the rest room where everybody went to smoke. You could hardly breathe in there."

"You have to try different things, and not just give up if you need to make a switch in what you're doing."

One nurse, when told by a colleague to "do that" (pump her milk) in the women's restroom, replied: "I am sure that you do not prepare your meals in the bathroom and my baby does not want me to prepare hers there either."

In this chapter we will present a number of breastfeeding strategies that have worked for other mothers. The one you devise will probably not be an exact copy of any of these methods, nor will your plan work the same for you every single day. It is extremely important to stay flexible.

The chapter is divided into sections that describe particular work situations and strategies other women have found successful in those circumstances. The categories are:

    I. FULL-TIME JOBS
   II. PART-TIME JOBS
  III. BABY BROUGHT TO YOU DURING WORKING HOURS
  IV. YOU GO TO BABY DURING WORKING HOURS
   V. BABY COMES TO WORK WITH YOU
  VI. TRAVELING

Included in most of the sections are "Problems" you might encounter with these methods and suggestions for "What to Do." Stories and comments from women who have used these strategies follow each section.

I. FULL-TIME JOBS

1. No Flexibility in Break Times

You have a specified time for breaks and lunch. This category may include occupations such as office work, industry, schoolteaching, construction.

- Breastfeed before leaving for work (allow enough time for a complete, relaxed feeding).
- Express milk on first break.
- Leave lunch open, unless your morning expression was not complete.
- Express milk on second break.
- Breastfeed the baby right away after work.
- Breastfeed as often as the baby wants in the evenings.
- Encourage night feedings (this will tend to reduce the feedings needed the next day).
- Breastfeed only (no bottles) on days off to rebuild supply.

Or you can . . .
- Breastfeed before leaving for work.
- Express milk on both breaks and at lunch.
- Breastfeed all feedings when at home.

Or you can . . .
- Breastfeed before leaving for work.
- Express remaining milk after you feed the baby.
- Express milk during your lunch break.
- Breastfeed all feedings when at home.

Or you can . . .
- Provide formula for missed feedings.
- Breastfeed all feedings when at home.

PROBLEM:

Your baby does not want to breastfeed in the morning before work.

What to Do:

Express your milk; don't force her to eat. Add this additional milk to the supply provided for that day because your baby may be hungrier later on. Note: If you don't express, you'll be uncomfortable at work.

PROBLEM:

You cannot always express successfully on your rigid break schedule.

What to Do:

• Ask your supervisor for flexible breaks, temporarily, until you wean your baby.
• Ask if you can take a shorter lunch or dinner break in exchange for slightly longer midday breaks.
• Contact your union representative for assistance in communicating your needs.
• Revise your breastfeeding strategy.
• Change jobs.

PROBLEM:

How much milk should you express?

What to Do:

• Experiment with one feeding by expressing milk and measuring the amount your baby takes.
• Ask the caregiver to keep track of the amount the baby consumes.

PROBLEM:

Your employer will not allow you to express at work or you do not have time to express at work.

What to Do:

- At home, breastfeed your baby on one breast, then use the other breast to express milk for the next day's missed feedings. (Alternate breasts each time you do this in order to maintain milk supply.)
- Go ahead and express your milk; what you do in the women's lounge is your privilege.
- Realize that his open lack of support places stress on you and may make expression more difficult. Use relaxation techniques (deep breathing, think about your baby, close your eyes).
- Consider using formula during the day and breastfeed frequently in the evenings, at night, and on weekends to keep up your supply.
- Talk with personnel, your union representative, or seek legal advice.
- Find a job that has a more supportive environment.

PROBLEM:

Where can you go to express milk, and where can you store it?

What to Do:

See Chapter Four, "Collecting and Storing Your Milk" and "Where to Pump Your Milk."

[Erica J. works on an assembly line. Although she is on flextime (she can arrive at work anytime between 7:00 A.M. and 8:30 A.M., and leaves after eight hours), her breaks during the day are fixed and only ten minutes each. Her lunch break is thirty minutes. Erica went back to work when her son was six weeks old and breastfed for six months.]

"I decided not to pump. I fed Tom at seven in the morning and then tried to get home from work by four. I just didn't think there was enough time in my day to pump, or to try to go home and nurse at lunch. I asked the sitter not to feed him after one. Then I'd feed him right away at four o'clock and usually three more times during the evening. He didn't eat a lot at one time, but he ate quite often!

"I should have started earlier 'training' my body to not make milk during the day. I waited until three days before I was supposed to go back to work; I should have started ten days or two weeks before that. I had enough milk for three kids at least, and it was real uncomfortable that first week back at work—readjusting to him not nursing during the day.

"The first day I practiced, I nursed Tom in the morning and then said, okay, I'm not nursing again until four. I soaked through three bath towels, and finally just lay in bed leaking. I should have started out skipping every other feeding rather than going cold turkey like I did.

"When I got back to work, it was hard. Toward the afternoon if I bumped anything, I'd leak. In fact, one day I had to stay until four-thirty. I accidentally bumped myself and it hurt terribly, and I leaked all over the place. I had soaked through my entire pad, so I had to go to the rest room and dry off with paper towels. As the baby got older, I didn't have as much trouble with leakage. The first two weeks were the worst."

2. Flexible Break Times

You can take your break and go to lunch at your own discretion (within reasonable limits).

- Breastfeed before going to work.
- Express your milk two to three times a day, when you feel full or your milk lets down.
- Breastfeed all feedings at home.

Or you can . . .
- Provide formula for missed feedings.
- Breastfeed all feedings when at home.

PROBLEM:

You can't always leave your job assignment when your breasts are full or your milk lets down.

What to Do:

• Wear breast shells or milk cups during the times you ordinarily let down.
• Talk with your employer and explain that you won't be dashing off forever—just until your baby gets a little older.
• When you do have time to express, make sure you empty your breasts completely.

[Allison G., a full-time office worker, breastfed and worked for three and a half months.]

"I tried at first to express my milk at the same time every day, but that doesn't always work if you're on the phone or you have a meeting. So I just left it up to my own body to tell me when I needed to express. And it usually came between ten-thirty and eleven (I would have fed her at six in the morning). I got a lot of milk out—six or seven ounces at that time. In the afternoon I'd pump at about three o'clock, and I didn't get quite as much, about three to four ounces. So I realized that whatever I would express during my workday was not going to be enough for Jill's feedings during the time I was at work. So I had to start supplementing. It was really trial and error. Some days she didn't want any more, and some days she'd be extra hungry so the formula helped out.

"It's not that you're doing something you're not supposed to be doing, but you are taking time away from your work. Feeling that way, plus the pace of the job, caused my milk supply to run down a little bit during the day. But I'd come home and nurse her at night, and I'd have plenty of milk."

"After about a month, when I'd go into the little stall in the bathroom every morning at a certain time, everyone knew why and they didn't even bother to try to come in. They knew I was in there pumping away!"

3. A Job with Rotating Shifts

This can be a tricky situation, because you are not gone at the same time every day. However, you will be at home some days and can breastfeed frequently to keep up your supply.

When working the day shift . . .
• Breastfeed before going to work.
• Express milk during breaks and at lunch.
• Breastfeed all other feedings at home.

When working the night shift . . .
• Breastfeed during the day.
• Express and save any excess milk after feedings.
• Breastfeed before leaving for work.
• Express milk once during the night (more if you become engorged, or if time permits).

Or you can . . .
• Provide formula for missed feedings.
• Breastfeed all feedings when at home.

PROBLEM:
Sometimes shifts are structed to be ten to twelve hours long.

What to Do:
• Plan at least three breaks for expression.
• Breastfeed frequently when at home.
• Arrange to leave work to go home and breastfeed.

PROBLEM:
Finding the time and place to express is difficult.

What to Do:
- Switch to a less demanding duty (i.e., work in outpatient services rather than intensive care) until the baby is older.
- For more privacy, express in a lounge or quiet office rather than in the nursery expressing room.
- Arrange with coworkers to cover for you when you need to express.

[Ann M. worked and breastfed her baby for one month after returning to full-time pediatric nursing.]

"I was working twelve-hour shifts, rotating between days and nights. There wasn't a set, consistent pattern. I pumped at work, but if there wasn't enough she got some formula. I pumped only once during the twelve hours. I started losing my milk supply, and after a while she didn't want to nurse as much—she was just as happy with the formula.

"I really needed to pump twice at work. But I couldn't because of the scheduling—you never know when you're going to be taking care of a sick infant. And even though my baby is more important to me personally, on the job I had a responsibility and there were times when I just could not leave."

II. PART-TIME JOBS

Many working/breastfeeding mothers return to work on a part-time basis until their babies are older. When working part-time, you can scale down the strategies suggested for a full-time schedule. The problems and solutions will be similar to those described under "Full-Time Jobs."

1. A Four-Hour Shift

- Breastfeed as close to your departure time as possible.
- Express milk during your break.
- Breastfeed at all other feedings.

If your child is older and taking fewer feedings, you may be able to get by without expressing at work. Leave an emergency bottle with your caregiver.

2. Two or Three Eight-Hour Days

- Use strategies for full-time schedule. On your days off, breastfeed all feedings.

Or you can . . .
- Breastfeed when you are at home and provide formula for missed feedings.

[Michelle I. works two eight-hour days for the public health department.]

"I breastfed Kyle before work, he got formula when I was at work, and I breastfed when I got home. I did that for the two days I was working, and when I wasn't working, I breastfed the whole time. It didn't bother my supply at all. It was amazing—I had the right amount of milk all the time. But he was about six months and was getting some solid foods. I had that same routine for fifteen months and it worked out just fine."

[Nan S. is a mechanical engineer who works for a computer manufacturer. When her daughter was twelve weeks old, she returned to work half-time, then resumed a full-time schedule at sixteen weeks.]

"When I went back to work part time she was sleeping through the night. I'd get up about six and feed her as close to seven as I could. I tried to get her good and full. My husband took her to the sitter at about seven-thirty, and I'd try to go to work as soon as I could after that. The sitter would usually give her two ounces of breastmilk (I had frozen bottles). At eleven-thirty I would run over and pick her up and go home and feed her.

"Many times I'd express my milk in the morning before I fed her. When I went back full time the sitter gave her a bottle in the morning, and between eleven-thirty and twelve I'd go over and spend my lunch hour with her and feed her. The sitter gave her a bottle in the afternoon, and then I'd pick her up at five and feed her right away. At first I tried to supply two bottles of breastmilk, but that got too hectic, so we used formula.

"I'd pack a lunch the night before and eat it at the sitter's, either while I was nursing or playing with her. She ate so fast that I had a good half hour to play with her. That was wonderful. I didn't pump at work. To get in the eight hours is tough, and pumping a couple times a day would have taken another half hour out of the day. I'd rather spend that time with her. I did have to express milk some afternoons in the bathroom when she didn't want to eat at lunchtime."

III. BABY BROUGHT TO YOU DURING WORKING HOURS

The women who can breastfeed during the workday usually have a caregiver, a relative or good friend who lives nearby. Perhaps your spouse can pick up the baby and bring her to your workplace or an at-home caregiver will agree to bring your baby to you.

1. No Flexibility in Lunch or Break Time

- The caregiver brings the baby at a prearranged time each day.
- You meet in a quiet, private place: empty room, conference room, your office, women's lounge, locker room, the car, empty dressing room (retail job).
- Have an alternate place in case your prearranged room is occupied.
- Make sure your caregiver is a good driver, and insist that your baby be transported in a National Highway Traffic Safety Administration approved infant car seat, properly belted.

- Have your caregiver bring the baby in a taxi (admittedly, this takes a lot of money and is not an option for most women).

PROBLEM:
You are having trouble coordinating your supply with the nursing breaks.

What to Do:
- Wear breast shells or milk cups to collect milk.
- Go to the rest room and express just enough to relieve the engorgement.
- Discuss flexible breaks with your employer.
- Arrange trades with coworkers.

PROBLEM:
Your baby gets hungry before the scheduled nursing time.

What to Do:
- Have the caregiver delay the baby by giving her a pacifier or a little warm water.
- Discuss flexible breaks with your employer.
- Leave a bottle of breastmilk or formula for a snack.
- On days when the baby simply cannot wait, have the caregiver call you and you express your milk at that feeding.

PROBLEM:
Weather conditions make it impossible or unsafe for the baby to be brought to you.

What to Do:
- Express milk until you can resume your routine.
- Provide formula for missed feedings.

[Jane T. is a bank teller. While her breaks are not completely rigid, she must arrange them with other tellers, and thus adheres to a planned schedule. At eleven-thirty and at three, Jane's caregiver drives the baby to the bank (a ten-minute trip) and they meet in the rest room, where there is a couch.]

"You have to have a real supportive baby-sitter. And mine doesn't have any other children to care for; if she did, this would be hard—maybe impossible. The most difficult part is the timing. I mean, babies' stomachs aren't clocks. Usually Andy will wait for me, but sometimes the sitter calls and says, 'He's hungry *now.*' If it's early and he just can't wait, she gives him a bottle. I always keep three or four bags of breastmilk in her freezer as well as a supply of formula.

"Of course, if she has to give him a bottle, I use my break to pump instead. But that doesn't happen too often, and I'm glad. I'm not very good at pumping. Most of the time she can stall Andy by leaving early and driving around town until it's time to meet me at the bank. He likes riding in the car, and that calms him down. But can you imagine? This woman is a real jewel!"

2. Flexible Break Times

Here, the caregiver calls you when the baby is hungry and you arrange your meeting time and place.

PROBLEM:
The baby wants more feedings than you have breaks.

What to Do:
- Express extra milk during the evenings and on weekends, and leave it with the caregiver.
- Leave formula with the caregiver, but request that she use other techniques (pacifier or water) if it is close to the time of the scheduled breastfeeding.
- The baby's extra-hungry days are nature's way of building up your supply. If you can, express some milk to signal your body to beef up production.
- Don't worry. These extra-hungry days will be temporary.

[Peggy B. is a pediatric nurse whose mother brought her baby to the office for feedings.]

"I tried really hard to be careful not to leave my coworkers in the lurch. I tried to make sure everything I was supposed to do was done and that it was an appropriate time to take a break."

IV. YOU GO TO BABY DURING WORKING HOURS

You would manage this alternative in much the same way as you did above, but you travel instead of the baby.

- If your breaks are flexible, the caregiver calls you when the baby is hungry.
- If your breaks are rigid, handle as above under "No flexibility in break time."

Note: If you live far from your job, this method can still work for you if you find a caregiver close to your workplace.

PROBLEM:
You have time to go to the baby only during lunch.

What to Do:
- Breastfeed at lunch and express during your breaks.
- Have the caregiver give the baby breastmilk at other feedings.
- Don't rush the noontime nursing. Express any milk the baby does not take.
- Or you can give formula for the missed feedings, making sure you breastfeed frequently when at home.
- Breastfeed as soon after work as possible, and ask the caregiver not to feed the baby close to the time of your arrival.

PROBLEM:
The baby doesn't want to nurse when you do.

What to Do:
- Express milk in the afternoon. If your time is limited, express enough to relieve your discomfort.

[Susan Y., retail clerk.]

"When I went back to work full time, she had several days when she couldn't make up her mind if she wanted the bottle or me. She got a little fussy because the schedule had changed, and she didn't eat at lunch for a few days. I ended up having to express in the afternoon. But eventually we got on a pretty good schedule, and I fed her every day at about eleven-thirty."

[Rita O. is a teacher who returned to work when her son was three months old.]

"I went to the baby-sitter's and nursed at noon. I supplemented Ian with water and juice in bottles. I breastfed him at eight and then went to the sitter's at about twelve-thirty. I'd be off at four, so I'd get to him again then. But by four my breasts would be really sore and burning.

"The sitter was two blocks away. I really liked that. I'd leave my car there in the morning, walk to school, and then walk back and forth again at lunch. I'd walk about a mile every day. It was excellent for getting back in shape after the pregnancy. That plus the nursing just burned the calories, and it seemed no time before the added weight was gone.

"Teachers do have noon duties. Most of the teachers were real supportive. There were two of us breastfeeding. One woman who had never had a baby did complain about it and felt it was unfair that we could get out of that noon duty. But two or three others had liked breastfeeding so much that they traded duties with us. We had recess duties and morning duties, and they took our noon duties. Anyone who had breastfed or had a child was very supportive."

* * *

[Doris P., who nursed her son for four months, is an assistant product manager for a major consumer-goods corporation.]

When Doris first went back to work she went home for lunch each day, about a twenty-minute drive, to breastfeed. She didn't pump at work, and her baby was given a bottle of formula in the afternoon. After a while, the noontime arrangement became too difficult to keep up, so she discontinued breastfeeding at that time but continued to nurse in the mornings and evenings. "I still went home at lunch but didn't breastfeed. It got to be too much of a hassle. I needed to fix my lunch and eat, and there just wasn't enough time. And sometimes I'd get caught in meetings and not make it home before he needed to be fed."

Doris describes her son Blake as "easygoing" about taking a bottle. When she began to eliminate breastfeedings, it was no problem for her son, and because the change was gradual, she experienced no discomfort or engorgement. "We just sort of went from four bottles to three to two."

When Blake was six months old, Doris went on a business trip, and the demanding schedule she had while she was away made pumping almost impossible. "It was a drag, trying to find places to pump, and needing to pump when I was supposed to be in meetings, and coming back to my room at night and having to pump." Because her job required some travel each month, she decided at this point to wean. "It was real hard to give up the breastfeeding, but I knew I had given him six good months, and that was all I could do. Breastfeeding is wonderful, but you don't need to break your back to do it. You do what you can."

[Mary L., office worker.]

"My mother never nursed a baby, and she will be the first to tell you that a breastfed baby is the worst baby to sit for— that bottle-fed babies are much easier, they sleep longer, they're not as fussy. But she was very willing to help me. If I was fifteen minutes late, she'd be walking the floors and pacifying him because she realized how much I wanted to continue with it. She made the extra effort to do all those things so that when I came home the baby was ready to nurse."

[Zoe W. is an engineer. Most of her coworkers are men.]

"Most of them think it's really neat. They see me leave at lunch and I've usually been going about a thousand miles an hour and upset about something. I go over there and play with her and come back completely relaxed and sometimes resolve problems a lot better. That is such a good break."

[Kay L. is a bank officer in a metropolitan area. Though her drive to work takes about fifty minutes, she found a caregiver only two minutes from her office. At noon, Kay goes to the caregiver's home to breastfeed.]

"The thought of a four-month-old baby in a long commute situation bothers me. But it doesn't bother her at all. She sleeps most of the time and is very content."

V. BABY COMES TO WORK WITH YOU

To bring your baby to work, you need a setting that is highly adaptable, coworkers who are 100 percent supportive, and the type of job that is interruptable. If you can get your work done, this situation can be ideal for breastfeeding and being close to your baby. If your job is conducive to this arrangement only part of the time, you can combine strategies: Bring the baby with you on days when you can juggle both her and your job; leave her with a caregiver and express milk on the days when you do not have the time to care for her. For this, you will need a flexible caregiver, perhaps a child-care home where you can leave your baby whenever you wish, or an exceptional family member who is willing to care for your child at a moment's notice.

Do not take your baby to work if you have to leave her unattended even for a short period of time.

PROBLEM:

Are your coworkers tolerant of children and supportive of your plan?

What to Do:
- Talk with each person individually before you make your decision.
- If you get a negative response, you may want to reconsider.
- Or ask your coworkers for suggestions about how you can make this plan work. Establish ground rules that you agree to abide by.
- Don't plan to use your coworkers to care for your baby if you are called away or get tied up. If someone really wants to help, that's fine, but don't count on them or build them into your plan. Make sure you can handle the situation on your own, and regard any helping hands as special bonuses.

PROBLEM:

Concentrating on your work and trying to watch your baby.

What to Do:
- Set up a portable crib, playpen, or sleep/play area near your desk or work assignment. Leave this setup at work.
- Keep a supply of safe toys in the baby's crib and another bag of toys to rotate for variety.
- Tie toys to the crib with short strips of fabric so you don't have to fetch them. Do not use string or rope, and keep the length of the strips short so the baby will not get tangled.
- Plan your work around your baby's schedule. Do jobs that require concentration during nap time.
- Use a backpack or soft baby carrier.

[Monica D. shares an office with a mother who brings her baby to work.]

"A lot of the times if it was annoying or distracting to me, I could go someplace else to do work. Sometimes I took care of the baby. I like babies, and if Renee was on the phone or was gone and the baby started fussing, I'd go over and talk to her or pick her up. But I didn't let it interfere with my work.

"At the time there was one woman in the office who was very offended by breastfeeding in public. She found it very offensive that Renee would nurse at meetings and felt that it was distracting—that people were paying more attention to the baby than to the agenda of the meetings. The majority of the people got used to the idea, and the baby was just part of the group and no focal point. But for a couple of people it was an excuse not to work, to play with the baby instead.

"I remember one meeting when Renee was nursing the baby and reached for some papers in the center of the table and leaked milk all over the papers belonging to the one woman who had always been very openly negative about her breastfeeding. I suppose she could have gotten very angry and stormed out, but she just got a napkin and wiped the papers off. It was an all-women meeting, and the rest of us just chuckled about it, but the look on her face was priceless! I guess the moral here is to be very careful about whose papers you leak on!

"Unfortunately, the woman who was offended talked to everybody else but never talked to Renee about it. I think you should talk to everybody and get their feelings. If you know that there are people who are offended by it, you could make it a point not to breastfeed when they're around. If you have a situation like ours, where you share an office, that takes even more preparation—working out a mutual agreement for those situations where it might become a distraction. In our situation, it worked out really well."

[Joyce F. works with an all-female staff in an office of Planned Parenthood. She brought her daughter Bridget to work with her for the first six months and continued breastfeeding until Bridget was twenty-two months old.]

"My day started at nine. My job was real varied as to what I'd do from day to day. I had a private office with a couch, so that made it really handy. I brought toys in and kept a bag of toys at the office so she'd have some things to watch, and I brought music so she'd have those kinds of stimuli.

"If I found myself on a long-distance phone call and she got fussy, there always seemed to be someone who'd run in and pick her up and take her out and walk her around. If I needed some time, or I needed to talk to a patient, there was always a staff member who was real willing to take her for a few minutes.

"When she was about four months old, I put Bridget in a backpack and carried her all over if I had to do inventory or make copies and go up and down the stairs. She liked that— she was old enough to look around and she enjoyed being out and seeing people. She's never had a fear of strangers, and I think that's from being around lots of different people at work.

"If I had a meeting we'd put her on a blanket on the floor. I never heard anyone make any comments. She'd nurse, and I'd go change diapers and come back and we'd continue on.

"You learn to breastfeed and write a letter at the same time. If I had a pile of writing or reading to do, I'd do those things during feeding time. Then I'd do things that involved being up and walking around when she was awake, and I'd take her with me. Sometimes I'd sit on the floor to do projects so I could talk to her and give her toys.

"I planned a lot before Bridget was born, getting ahead on work and things that would be due. I decided maybe I'm not going to be my most productive in these few months that she's there, but I'm going to be well prepared before she gets here. And I brought work home if I didn't finish.

"You might not end work right when you walk out the door, but you have the baby with you all that time. It was a real easy trade-off for me. It would be very, very hard if you didn't have some flexibility in the job, or if you had a job where you were required to do things at certain times, if you had to be places, or if you had letters to get out at a certain time. Because if that's the baby's fussy time, that's the fussy time!

"Once a restaurant gave me a real problem about bringing the baby there for a business lunch. I said, 'I bring her to work; why can't I bring her to a restaurant?' They said they didn't have high chairs or booster seats. I said she was an infant, but they said they 'didn't encourage children.' So I called another restaurant and was given a huge booth and lots of attention and concern.

"There were definitely some people I met who were appalled by what I was doing. But you find that even if you're walking in a shopping mall and stop to breastfeed on a bench. Some people will ask if there is anything they can do to help; other people look at you as if you are being obscene."

VI. TRAVELING

Breastfeeding and traveling is probably the most difficult arrangement to manage. Your strategy will depend on how long you're gone each time, whether or not the baby (and in many instances a caregiver) can travel with you, and how efficient your pumping techniques are.

1. Daytime Travel; Home at Night

- Manage as you would on a regular eight-hour schedule (see suggestions under "Full-time Jobs").
- Locate places where you can express milk (the office to which you travel, your car, women's lounges).
- Carry your milk-storage system with you.
- Express and discard milk if no portable storage system is possible.
- Provide breastmilk or formula for the baby in your absence.

- Practice pumping techniques; you will need to be able to let down and express milk easily in a variety of settings.
- Breastfeed frequently when at home and on weekends.

Or you can . . .
- Take your baby with you.

[Nancy W. was required to attend an out-of-town meeting twice a month and one overnight trip each month.]

"I had a really hard time pumping—getting myself to let down. By the end of the day I'd be really engorged, so full I'd bounce home.

"It helped when my husband drove with me and we took the baby. He did other things while I went to the meeting. I brought Alan to the meeting and he hung out on the floor and was just fine. But that only worked when my husband was free. Later, I went by myself and took Alan. I found a baby-sitter there by talking to friends, so I didn't need to take him to the meetings."

2. Overnight Travel

- Take a caregiver or family member with you.
- If the baby is left at home, express milk when you can, preferably on the same schedule you ordinarily express or breastfeed.
- Discard expressed milk unless you can obtain or carry a storage system that will stay as cold as a refrigerator for forty-eight hours.
- Discard refrigerated milk after forty-eight hours, or whenever you have concerns that the milk has been inadequately refrigerated.
- Provide breastmilk or formula for the baby in your absence.
- Nurse frequently when you return home.

[Becky K. took her mother and two children to a three-day conference.]

"We stayed in the motel where the conference was being held. I'd nurse the baby and run down to the meetings, and in between on breaks I'd run up and nurse, and my mother would call room service and have a sandwich waiting for me. It worked well. We took a stroller so she could go on walks. Only a grandma would volunteer to do this!

"Everybody in the conference knew I had my baby upstairs. But very seldom in a conference do you meet for more than two and one half or three hours, and most conferences give you a thirty-minute break. So you have to be committed to running up and sitting down and nursing as soon as the meeting is over. But we had bottles of formula just in case.

"The biggest obstacle is money. When you're traveling and need to take someone with you, you have her air travel and room and food to think about. I was lucky because my father offered to pay for my mother's expenses. And she was in a position where she was free and could leave for three days."

3. Extended Travel (More Than a Few Days)

- Bring the baby and a caregiver with you.
- If the baby is left at home, express milk on a regular routine.
- Discard expressed milk, unless you can freeze it properly and transport it home at a temperature of zero degrees Fahrenheit.
- Nurse frequently when you get home.
- Try to plan your trip so that you have a weekend or a couple of days off to rebuild your supply of milk.

PROBLEM:
Your milk supply decreases.

What to Do:
- Express as often as you would at home.
- Empty your breasts completely; if you can't do this, express more often.

PROBLEM:
Your schedule is too demanding to allow consistent, complete milk expression.

What to Do:
- Organize meetings and duties around the times you ordinarily need to express.

Or . . .
- Express just enough to relieve engorgement and discomfort. Then, when you get home, breastfeed full time and express any surplus milk to rebuild your supply.

Note: The time it takes to rebuild your supply will be about the same as the time you were not breastfeeding. If you are gone for forty-eight hours, it will take about forty-eight hours to regain your supply. If you take two weeks off, it will take two weeks of very diligent breastfeeding to rebuild your supply.

[Carol U. is an electrical engineer in a large electronics corporation. She had been back to work for one week when she was asked to travel to Japan for seven days. Her baby was twelve weeks old.]

"The advice I got from other people was interesting. For example, they suggested: Don't work at all; don't go on the trip; go on the trip and take the baby; go on the trip and take my husband; insist that the company pay for all our expenses. My response was: Given that I am going on the trip and I'm not taking the baby or my husband, Now what do I do? I was most concerned about keeping up my milk supply while I was gone. I eventually got some tips on how to use the breast pump and get my let-down reflex to work, because I'd always had trouble with that."

For a couple of weeks before the trip, Carol practiced with the pump. She used techniques for breast massage and also a warm cloth to assist the let-down. Eventually she became proficient with the pump, and these extra pumpings also increased her milk supply so that she was able to save and freeze breastmilk. By the time she left, she had saved about 50 percent of the amount her baby would need while she was away. Formula was alternated with the breastmilk.

Carol's regular baby-sitter cared for her baby during the day, and her husband willingly took over the rest of the time. Then came the job of maintaining her supply while she was away.

"I explained to the people who were arranging our meetings, and also to my boss, that I needed to be able to excuse myself at least once, maybe twice, during the day, for thirty to forty minutes at a time. My boss said that would be fine.

"The flight was eleven hours, and pumping on a plane is not a good time. I had to go into the bathroom, because I couldn't imagine myself sitting next to my boss and pumping milk. In the bathroom it was sort of like sitting in an outhouse for forty-five minutes. And when you hit air turbulence, there's nothing to hold you down. It's just not conducive to pumping at all. I had to throw the milk away. The first time I almost cried—it seemed like such a waste. And I wondered what everyone was thinking when they walked to the back of the plane, because you can hear those pumps a mile away!

"In Japan, I expressed about every four hours during the day, and once or twice during the evening. The worst of it was that there was no place to go. Not many Japanese women work, and the rest-room facilities were only a little better than they were on the plane. There is no place to sit down, because the toilets are more like a hole in the floor. I'd be standing there with no place to hang my coat or my purse, and this pump and all my stuff crammed in there. Then I had a dress on, which I had to unbutton, and I'd just pray that the whole thing wouldn't dump all over me. After three days of that, I slowed down to three, maybe four pumpings a day, and by the time I got home my supply had definitely decreased.

"When I got off the plane, my baby had no idea who I was, but that was okay with me because my doctor had told me to expect that. I nursed right away and he just latched right on and knew exactly what to do. I gave him some supplements until my milk supply built back up."

Carol had arranged with her boss to take several days off after the trip. She used this time to rest, to replenish her milk supply, and to spend some time with her son.

"The whole thing was more than I had anticipated, but it worked out okay. I was very determined. And by contrast, the trip to Japan made the idea of going back to work seem simple!"

A GREAT PLACE FOR MOTHERS: ONE COMPANY'S STORY

At Beth Israel Hospital in Boston, new mothers are not only supported, they are encouraged to breastfeed and given lots of real help as they make the transition back to work. Called The Breastfeeding Support Program, this pioneering plan was founded in 1987 by Sandra Reed Sweezy, nurse and breastfeeding expert, who noticed that new mothers on the hospital staff were searching for private places to express milk, and also asking for a lot of help on how to continue breastfeeding after returning to work. Sweezy worked with the hospital administration to create a support system for these mothers.

In this program, a few weeks before her expected return to work, a new mother can call in and receive a telephone consultation. This consultation allows her to start planning her breastfeeding strategy and to get answers to questions on topics such as storing milk, child care, and introducing a bottle.

The mother is also invited to come into the hospital, with the baby, for some one-on-one guidance with a breastfeeding expert, to plan exactly how, when, and where she will express and store her milk. On her first day back to work, she again meets with a nurse consultant who demonstrates the use of the breast pump and stands by if she wants more assistance in using the pump for the first time. Later, follow-up help is available.

There are two locations where breastfeeding personnel at Beth Israel can find electric breast pumps. A pump for staff use only is located in a private examining room in the employee occupational health service wing. During off hours, when that area of the hospital is closed, personnel use the patient breast pumps on the obstetrical floor. For the program, Sweezy chose an electric breast pump, with a flexible flange and adaptability for bilateral pumping, to enhance long-term milk volume. Mothers can purchase their breast pump accessory kit right in the hospital's gift shop. The hospital provides a refrigerator/freezer used only for storing milk.

A study of the Beth Israel program mirrors other research on breastfeeding and working, which has shown that women who are able to express milk at missed feedings tend to breastfeed longer than those who do not. In an employee newsletter, Sweezy said: "Many women may choose not to breastfeed their infant or may prematurely wean their infant because they believe they have no other choice. With this program, women now have a choice."

7

Women in Unusual Job Situations

"At lunch I go out of the office and there are a million things on my mind—there are presentations and things breaking—but as soon as I get to the sitter's it all goes out of my mind. I don't think of anything but my little girl until I go back to work. It's a great break."

"If you have somebody you know who has done it, it really helps a lot. If you know it's happened before, there's a good chance you can make it happen, too."

"I can't count the number of times women asked me to go out and have a beer after work, and I couldn't go. But I wanted to go. It's hard. You have to be pretty darn determined and not very selfish."

"I've worn plenty of essence of spit-up back to work after lunch, but they get used to me."

In this chapter, we'll tell the stories of women who are in work or life situations that call for particularly creative breastfeeding strategies.

Single Parent

[Wendy N. is a twenty-three-year-old single mother who held two different jobs during the fourteen months she nursed her daughter. When Laurel was a few weeks old, Wendy resumed her work as a radio announcer for a small-town radio station, and Wendy's mother brought the baby to the station for meals. They weren't exactly a conventional song-and-dance routine, but it wasn't unusual to find Laurel happily breastfeeding while Wendy spun platters and made announcements.]

"She was the greatest," says Wendy. "I'd turn the mike on and start talking, and when she was done nursing she never cried." Occasionally, says Wendy, Laurel gurgled a remark of her own, bringing letters and calls from delighted listeners.

Wendy had known and worked for the owner of the station for a number of years and had no difficulty when she decided to bring her baby into her work life. "It was just assumed I'd do it," she says, "so his reaction was 'of course, what else?' It was a family-run station, and I was just like one of the family. The only problem was some embarrassment if my boss or his brother walked in on me while I was nursing."

When Laurel was nine months old, Wendy moved to another town and started an 8:00–5:00 job as a retail store manager. At first she went to the baby during her lunch hour to breastfeed. But that arrangement didn't work well.

"She wanted to do what she wanted to do. My lunch hour was at twelve and she wasn't always hungry at twelve. Trying to get her to fit into my schedule was real difficult. So we introduced the bottle [formula] and she took it just fine. After that, I nursed her in the morning, at night when I got home, and again before bedtime."

When she eliminated the noon feeding, Wendy was surprised that she did not experience any engorgement, and her milk supply stayed stable. "I think during the few weeks of trial and error at noontime my breasts adjusted to her not taking milk at noon, and tapered off just right. I had plenty of milk the other times."

To a single, working mother like Wendy, breastfeeding was significantly more economical, and also time-saving. "It's so easy to sit down and watch the news and nurse, than come home and try to fix bottles with her screaming and everything more hectic." And for Wendy, breastfeeding was more than a method for feeding and nurturing her baby; it was a way she got nurtured, too.

"As a single parent, I needed support and love and tenderness, and the baby gave that to me. Nursing supported *me.* And I felt that she needed twice as much from me, and nursing also provided that. My sitter is always telling me that Laurel is such a loving child. She takes care of the other babies and gives lots of hugs and kisses. I'm sure this has something to do with nursing."

Engineer, Full Time

[Sandra T. breastfeeds and works as a technical engineer for a large manufacturing company. She leaves her workplace at noon and travels two miles to her caregiver's for the noon feeding. Sandra's midmorning and afternoon breaks are only ten minutes, too short for her to express and save milk. For these feedings, Jessica receives formula at the caregiver's. Sandra breastfeeds in the mornings, after work, and at bedtime. At four months, Jessica was sleeping through the night. At six months she received solids once every evening.]

Sandra describes her job as highly stressful because of constant project deadlines and "high visibility" by upper management. She does, however, work on a flex-time schedule— she can go to work anytime between 6:00 A.M. and 8:30 A.M., and may leave when she has completed eight hours.

Sandra's caregiver is also a nursing mother, and consequently very supportive of her breastfeeding routine. "I take my lunch and put it in her refrigerator in the morning, then at lunch we sit and talk and nurse our babies. It's been a real good relationship for both of us."

Sometimes Jessica is not hungry at noon. But even if she eats very little, she usually takes enough to prevent Sandra from becoming engorged later in the day. If Sandra needs to work overtime, she leaves the workplace to breastfeed and returns to begin the overtime. This is fine with her supervisor.

"I don't have any free time. I spend every lunch hour feeding her and have to come home immediately after work to feed her. I don't go out on 'ladies' night out' the way some ladies do. I have to feed her every morning, and if she wakes up and needs feeding at night, I am the one who does it, not my husband."

But the positives far outnumber the negatives, Sandra says.

"I think it's really important when you're going back to work. I really enjoy the closeness Jessie and I have shared during the nursing relationship. And it's something that nobody else can do for her—anybody can give her a bottle but only her mommy can nurse her. When she smiles up at me it makes me feel really good. It's a time when I can stop everything that's going on in my world and just enjoy my baby. Ladies' night out will still be around when she's weaned."

Notes:

- If Sandra becomes engorged, she could use the short break to express just enough milk to relieve the discomfort, until the baby gets a bit older and/or the milk supply adjusts to the new routine.
- If the baby refuses to nurse at the noontime feeding, Sandra could use that time to express milk and store it at the caregiver's.

Bank Officer Turned Freelancer

[When Joyce W. learned she was pregnant, she was sure about two things: She wanted to stay home with her baby for four months, and she wanted to continue her career as manager of commercial marketing for a large Chicago bank-holding company. The solution seemed logical enough: Work at home for the first four months.]

"In talking with my manager, the vice-president of marketing [also a woman], we came up with the idea that I could essentially do work at home for the company and perform the same function I did in my job, so that my position could continue. As she put it, 'There's nothing that ties you to this building, other than the fact that everyone normally comes in here to go to work.' It was very easy to perform the job I had at home.

"But when we took the idea to personnel, they were up in arms, worried about policy and setting precedents. Then we came up with the idea of my resigning from the company and becoming a freelancer. We had an informal, though written, agreement that when I came back, I would be rehired for the same position."

One hitch in this arrangement was that Joyce had to give up her benefit package during the time she was freelancing. However, in the written agreement, all of her benefits and retirement would be reinstated at no penalty when she returned full time. (Luckily, Joyce was covered under her husband's health policy during the months she freelanced. Otherwise, this could have been a serious drawback to the plan.)

Both Joyce and her manager were aware that they were breaking new ground in creating this particular work arrangement. "It was an attempt to find some kind of workable situation for women who want to work and have a family as well.

"I essentially did the same job, but I did it in my home. I stopped in at the office once each week to check in, although I didn't stay long, because I always had my baby with me."

Joyce was paid an hourly wage that was based on her annual salary. "I logged hours, wrote down what project I was working on and submitted it." Joyce used the clerical services at the bank but was not compensated for her phone expenses and mileage. She was allowed to submit up to forty hours per week of freelance work.

She laughs. "I thought it would be no problem at all to work forty hours a week—I thought babies slept all day long. As it turned out, if I got a chunk of five hours at a time, that was a real big stretch! I ended up working about twenty hours a week. I mostly worked when Kerry napped and early in the morning. I had a baby swing, and if I wound it three times, that was forty-five minutes." Joyce breastfed her son on demand.

When the four months were over, Joyce worked in the afternoons for a couple of weeks to ease the adjustment for her and her baby. She pumped milk and left a bottle with the caregiver, and by this time Kerry was down to four feedings a day.

When Joyce returned to work full time, she went to the caregiver's for the noontime feedings (about a two-minute drive), and left bottles of breastmilk for the missed morning feedings. She pumped at work and stored the breastmilk in a refrigerator there. Usually her son was ready to eat when his mother arrived at noon, and if he got hungry earlier, the caregiver pacified him by holding and walking him.

As far as the response from other supervisors and coworkers, Joyce never worried about her pumping or breastfeeding arrangement.

"As long as it didn't interfere with my work, I felt I had a perfect right to go there. It never occurred to me that there would be any problem with this. Women often get a bum rap in the business world, and unless things change they'll continue to. People have to be more flexible, either that or rule out a big part of the possible work force.

"The president of our company was curious about what was going on, but he knew I was nursing in the afternoon, and he thought it was great. I think you need to work out a reasonable solution in your own mind and present it to your manager. If you come with the problem and the solution at the same time, it can probably work out, as far as working and breastfeeding or expressing milk. As for freelancing at home, that was a tough one, and I felt very lucky to be able to get that.

"It is special treatment, but having a baby is pretty special and you do have to have special treatment. It's not like you can pretend you can resume the work style of every other man in the office. There seems to be a lot of talk about 'giving special treatment' and having to 'break rules,' as if that's unjust, when the circumstance is extraordinary to begin with. It's not that men are saying don't have kids, but a lot of men don't seem to be able to accept having to treat breastfeeding women differently."

Self-Employed, Works Out of Home

["Opening night" for Rosemary S. came nearly on the heels of the cesarean birth of her daughter, Joy. Three months after her daughter was born, Rosemary was scheduled to open a movie theater. Her juggling act began right away, in her home office, as she finalized the plans to launch her business. New businesses take time and energy, and Rosemary's was no exception. Although the doctor had recommended she take some time off, there simply wasn't any time to spare.]

"Before we opened the theater, I had a teenager come to the house if I had to go out. All the other time I tried to work when she was sleeping, and of course when she was little she slept a lot. I worked on her schedule. If she got up, I just put my work aside. That worked out pretty well, but sometimes I'd be in the middle of something and didn't want to quit."

Though in one sense her work schedule was flexible, being self-employed brought its own set of pressures. Rosemary started back to work within two weeks. "There was so much to do. When you're managing your own business, the work is never done. I felt pressure to do the work rather than play with the baby or take a nap or do the laundry. I would say that during that time I worked forty to fifty hours a week.

"Once the theater opened I had to be down there a lot of the time, even though I still kept my office in my home. I took Joy to a day-care center anywhere between eight-thirty and ten-thirty in the morning. Sometimes it was pretty difficult because she was a fussy eater and didn't always want to nurse before I left her in the morning. Fortunately, the woman who kept her was close enough that I could go back over and try again in an hour or two."

Rosemary was usually able to pick up her daughter by four-thirty in the afternoon. After spending a few hours together, she took the baby back to the caregiver's and returned to the theater for the evening shift. Once a week it was necessary for Rosemary to stay until midnight. Joy was given formula for feedings when Rosemary was unable to get to the caregiver's to breastfeed.

"I never got very good at expressing milk. I found it to be too uncomfortable and too slow. And happily, the baby liked formula—it didn't seem to make much difference to her."

As for her schedule, Rosemary admits she "felt frantic for a while. It wasn't really the way I thought or hoped it would be. When we first started talking about the theater, I thought how much fun it would be. But I didn't have any concept of how much work it would take."

Rosemary had mastitis on the night of the theater's grand opening, which she believes was caused by a number of instances of engorgement from her erratic breastfeeding schedule. "And I was really exhausted, too. That didn't help."

After her daughter was weaned at eight months, Rosemary established a more predictable routine. Now Joy goes to day care at 9:30 and her mother returns at 5:00. Rosemary is not sure whether her life is less hectic or she is simply "getting better at it," but she does feel that the new schedule helps.

"For one thing, during the hours I'm with Joy, I'm *really*

with her. When I'm done working, I've learned to quit. I play with her and don't try to get her to entertain herself so I can get some more work done. We have dinner and we do the dishes or laundry, and we also take a bath together or go for a walk together—something that's fun. After she goes to bed, I do some more work, but I don't try to juggle both at one time anymore.

"If I were going to do it all over again, I'd take six months off, or have a job where I only worked about twelve hours a week."

Coal Miner

[When Donna L. was breastfeeding her baby she worked a mile underground in a Kentucky coal mine. Her job: keeping a coal belt running. Much of the time she worked by herself, but this was only one of the many ways in which she was alone. Donna was the only woman in the mine, and one of the first pregnant coal miners in the country.]

"I got up at four in the morning and would spend a couple of hours with my baby. I breastfed as long as she wanted to. Then at about six-thirty I'd go to work and take my pump with me. I used a hand pump. I would go underground, and at about ten o'clock or so my milk would let down and I'd pump my breasts. I'd keep my milk in my pump in my lunchbox and then take it home and put it in the freezer. When I got home at about three-thirty, I'd breastfeed her again, and then as often as she wanted."

For the first five months Rachael was exclusively breastfed. If she got thirsty in between feedings, she was happy with water. "We had a special communication," Donna says. "Rachael and I were very, very close. There was a fantastic bond. It was almost as if she understood the way we did things."

Donna did not worry about contamination from the heavy dust in the mine. The pump was never opened to the air, except at the flange where it contacted her breast. After pumping, she popped the milk into her lunchbox. Because the floor of the mine is cool, the milk stayed fresh without a need for ice or a thermos.

"Rachael's five years old now, and she's never really been sick—maybe a cold once in a while—but that's all. From the time she was born she grew normally and healthily."

Although Donna's job afforded her the privacy to express milk, her coworkers were aware of her midmorning pumpings. "The men had the funniest reactions. One day one of the guys opened my lunchbox and pulled out the milk and said, 'Uuugghh! You do that?' And I said, 'Yeah. Drink up. You'd probably like that stuff.' "

Being a pregnant miner, then a breastfeeding one, brought mixed reviews in the small town where Donna lived, but for the most part, the men in the mine were supportive. For almost three years Donna had been the only woman working with these men. "It was like we were brothers and sister," she says, adding, "but they'd never admit to that. But having me there brought about a lot of talk about babies and breastfeeding, conversations that men wouldn't normally have with each other. I had a lot of wonderful conversations. My being pregnant actually brought us closer.

"I worked underground until I was seven months pregnant. Talk about reactions! The breastfeeding was nothing compared to the fact that I was pregnant. When they first found out they'd say, you can't do this, you can't do that, you can't bend over, take it easy on the shoveling. If I didn't answer the phones they'd freak out and they'd come and check on me. We became very close."

As for the wives of the miners and the people in the community, "that was a whole other story," Donna says. "A lot of the time it was very upsetting. No one understood why a woman would go into a coal mine. There was a lot of admiration for the *men* who went underground because they worked hard and broke their backs, and when they came home from work they were pampered by the women. I mean, they'd been down there in the deep, dark mine all day. No woman could do this! People would take a look at me and say: '*You* do that? You're so little. Of course you don't *work*.' And that's what a lot of the men told their wives—that I wasn't there to work, that while they were breaking their backs, I was lying on mine."

Down in the mine, the men dropped the facade and were sincere. They told her: "Donna, you're a good worker. Don't let anyone kid you. You can outwork any of the men down here." But above ground, relationships were sometimes strained. "When you work with men for four years, and then walk into a room with their wives and sit down and start talking shop— you get some strange vibes. Some of the women became friends, but most of them stayed enemies. They thought I was having everybody's baby. They named my daughter Barbie, because the tunnel I worked in was called the Barbie seam."

For Donna, breastfeeding may have been the easiest of all the challenges she had to face.

"Breastfeeding is the most beautiful experience a woman could ever have. The ultimate. By not breastfeeding, women cheat themselves out of the best gift they'll ever get. If a woman is in an unusual job situation, there are hard times. But when it comes to breastfeeding your child, you can convince most people that it's very important. Hang in there, and hang tough. You'll never regret it."

8

Weaning

"It was harder weaning me than the baby," says Barbara N., a store manager who nursed her baby for fourteen months. "I enjoyed it so much I was not really willing to give it up."

"I didn't realize I was being so selfish about it until I got ready to wean," says Crystal J., whose son stopped breastfeeding at seventeen months. "I thought: 'I don't know if I want to do this. Are we still going to be a team?' But later I realized Joel and I were just as close a team. He can kiss me and hug me. There are just as many other good things that happen after breastfeeding."

When weaning happens naturally, it is usually a gradual process with little discomfort for you or your baby. Typically at around nine months, the baby becomes less interested in the breast. Sometimes she won't want to nurse, preferring to play or drink from a bottle or cup. At other times, you both might simply forget a feeding. Or you might miss a feeding and realize that the baby didn't mind at all. Before long, you are breastfeeding only once or twice a day, perhaps in the mornings and evenings. As you taper off, your milk supply gradually diminishes until eventually you aren't breastfeeding at all. During this period, which can last from a few weeks to several months, you will have days when your baby wants to nurse frequently again. Maybe she's teething, or under the weather, or needs a little extra mothering. Expect these regressions; they will be temporary. When you begin producing little, if any, milk, the baby is mostly interested in the comforting feeling of suckling and may want to have a few quick strolls down memory lane before moving on.

There are no "shoulds" about weaning. However, at about six months your baby will need more iron than your milk supplies, and iron-containing foods are often the first complementary source of nourishment. This is called mixed feeding, and the introduction of additional nutrients through solid foods need not interfere with your output of milk. Also at this age, your baby will be physiologically ready for chewing and learning how to eat from a spoon. Besides being a source of variety in foods, these activities are fun for the baby to master and can be used in place of some feedings. This gradual expansion of the baby's culinary world eases the adjustment to weaning for both of you.

Most of the women we talked with were not able to pinpoint an exact time when their babies were weaned. And though most of them were sorry to see the nursing relationship come to an end, they remember the process itself as easy and problem free.

When Karen E.'s son was a year old, he was down to a morning and evening feeding. Then he started sleeping later, and did not seem to mind missing that feeding, says Karen. "The last one Ted gave up was at night, and sometime after his first birthday he just turned his head away when I tried to feed him."

Once in a while after he was weaned, Ted would be fussy and want to nurse. "Sometimes I'd get home from work, and he'd go for it," Karen remembers. "Then I went on a business trip for several days, and that was about it. I did express milk while I was gone, but there wasn't much there. I was never engorged or uncomfortable."

At about six months, Sue R. noticed that her milk supply seemed to be decreasing. She was expressing once a day but only getting about three ounces by this time. "It didn't seem worth it to me to spend all that time expressing such a small amount—that was only a snack to the baby." Sue stopped pumping at work but continued breastfeeding mornings and evenings at home. Maggie was eating solids and enjoyed the variety in food.

Eventually Sue stopped the night feeding, because her husband wanted to feed Maggie before bed. At first she expressed breastmilk for this feeding, but she soon opted for the convenience of formula. Sue was happy to have the new free time. The morning feeding continued for a while longer, but Sue thinks her daughter felt obligated.

"It was like she thought: 'I guess I'm supposed to be doing this because my mom is offering it to me, but I'd really rather have the bottle.' When you're trying to get ready for work and you have this baby trying to make up her mind if she wants to nurse or not, you just don't have the time to sit around and wait for her decide. So I offered her a bottle, and if she wanted it, fine.

"It was almost like a mutual thing," says Sue. "I think I was burned out, and she was getting more from the bottle. It wasn't a really emotional, traumatic split. It was: 'Well, Mom, thanks; it's been fun.' "

The first thing to go will be your need to pump at work (yea!). You may have decided that your baby can get by with formula, cow's milk, juice, or solids at the caregiver's, with breastfeedings during the hours you are at home. If your baby is younger than nine months, some form of milk should constitute the majority of her food supply. If you are weaning before this age, you should use formula to meet her nutritional needs.

For a while, you may need to express just enough milk to relieve discomfort, but eventually you can eliminate workday pumpings altogether. (Hi, it's me—anybody want to go to lunch?) Your milk supply will begin to decline, and the process is under way. However, a morning and nighttime feeding can be maintained for some months and, if you desire, may continue beyond the second year.

Sometimes older babies and toddlers show no inclination to give up the breast, clinging tenaciously to a favorite feeding, perhaps at bedtime or in the morning, or demanding snacks anytime, anywhere. How you handle this is up to you, but unless you are terribly anxious to have breastfeeding over, you need not be concerned, nor do you need to take an abrupt no-more-breast stand. If you would rather your toddler didn't climb up onto your lap and unbutton your blouse in the middle of a dinner party, you certainly can make it clear that there are special times to nurse and this isn't one of them. Give lots of hugs and attention during this time, offer an alternative drink from a cup or bottle, and explain that you will nurse her later. Stall her whenever you can, but don't cut her off cold turkey, and allow her all the time she wants when she is nursing. Remember that only a few months ago you managed five or six feedings a day. One in the evening will cause little inconvenience and will ordinarily end of its own, very peaceful, accord.

Val H. recalls a few days when her daughter played with her, grabbing her nipple and yanking it back and forth. "I didn't think that was fun. She'd clamp down real hard and it hurt. I talked to my pediatrician, and he explained that it was a really pleasurable sensation for her—but, I had to let her know that was not what I was offering my breast for. If she wanted to play, I'd give her something to play with or chew. If she wanted to eat, she could nurse."

Kelly W.'s son weaned himself naturally at eighteen months. "I had pretty much dried up, I think, a month or two before he quit nursing. My breasts didn't seem to be filling up at all, and he cared less and less about it. When I did quit, he didn't care at all, and I wasn't sore." Kelly says she was sorry to give it up, but at this point her husband was putting some pressure on her to quit. "He thought the baby was way too big." Because the baby had been taking a bottle at the caregiver's, the transition from the breast to the bottle was very smooth.

Beverly R., who breastfed her baby for twenty-two months, admits that nursing an older child can be awkward. "So you go to pick them up at lunch, and you go to McDonald's and have a burger and fries, and then they ask, 'Can I nurse before you go back to work?' To many people this is outrageous."

When the baby is older and receiving other sources of nourishment, breastfeeding is often continued mostly for the emotional satisfaction it gives both mother and child. When you are working, this special time together is hard to give up, and it is often the mother who is last to be "weaned."

In the case of an older toddler who stubbornly insists on several feedings a day or gets very angry when the breast is not instantly available, there are some artful dodges you can try, suggests Karen Pryor in her book *Nursing Your Baby*. She cites rural Mexico, where mothers put chili powder on their breasts. The trick here is to act surprised and sorry when the baby encounters the unpleasant taste. In other parts of the world women use food coloring to tint their breasts or nipples, which is rather disconcerting to the child. Or you can plan a several-day trip away from your baby, giving her a chance to get along without breastfeeding for a while. In our interviews, we found women who tasted their milk in the later months of nursing and found it to be very salty, suggesting that nature may have its own mechanisms for making mother's milk less yummy as time goes on. Also, at about nine months the let-down reflex often wanes, and the baby begins to wean herself because she simply gets tired of waiting at longer and longer intervals for milk to come.

The circumstance most pertinent to working/breastfeeding women is the need to abruptly wean from the breast, when job pressures dictate, or when a long separation is expected. This can be difficult. It may take several feedings for the baby to accept the bottle, solids, or cup (what you substitute will depend on the baby's age). Sometimes babies refuse all liquids and will only take solids for a day or so.

Abrupt weaning, if the baby is only four to six weeks old, can cause engorgement, discomfort, or mastitis. Sometimes women experience "milk fever," a flu-like condition believed to be a result of milk being reabsorbed into the system. Milk fever lasts from three to four days. If you have to wean your baby abruptly, especially in the early weeks or months, you may be sad and possibly depressed. These feelings of loss and disappointment are natural and can be partly physical, a result of sudden hormonal changes from the cessation of lactation. You will need lots of support from people who care about you, and you will need to be very gentle on yourself. Remember that whatever time you spent breastfeeding is important— you got your baby off to the best possible start with the best possible food.

❧ 9

Special Tips for Fathers

You've made it through the first few weeks with your new baby. Ever so slightly, the pace begins to slacken and there are brief hints that life may eventually settle into some kind of a routine. You risk taking a deep breath.

Then your wife starts making plans to go back to work. Hopefully you've already had a number of discussions about her plan to continue breastfeeding. But as the time grows nearer, you may be struck by the enormity of jamming two full-time jobs—working and parenting—into one short day. The anxieties and concerns you feel are normal. It seems like too much for one person to do alone. The truth is, it is. But *two* can do it.

Women who successfully combine working and breast-feeding have the active and constant support of at least one other person—a husband, partner, mother, family member, or close friend. And those who have partners who become an integral part of the nursing team say they couldn't have survived without them.

Sure, you can't breastfeed the baby. But that hardly diminishes the part you play in how your baby is fed. Your active role in the care of your baby and your willingness to share all the demands of parenting are a big part of what makes breast-feeding possible. So in a very real sense, you are just as vital to your baby's nourishment as the person who is producing the milk.

"My husband has been extremely supportive," says Betsy R., a teacher who works and breastfeeds her son. "I couldn't have done it all without him."

Audrey G., also a teacher, says that one of the best things her husband does for her is to get up and take care of the baby on weekends so she can catch up on her rest. And when their son was three and a half months old, Audrey's husband took over the night feedings, giving the baby a bottle of formula. "That means in the morning I have a lot more milk, and if I have time to pump there is enough leftover."

Lindsay T.'s partner is a great help, especially in the morning. "He gets up, showers, and then brings the baby to me in bed. After I breastfeed her, I have so many things to do—for example, I have to eat a good breakfast, and I hurry to get to work early so I can get off early. So Rick changes her diaper, gets her dressed, packs her bag, and takes her to the sitter.

"The other night I worked late," Lindsay says. "When I got home I was so full and uncomfortable, and I worried that Rick had given her a bottle already. But he hadn't—he had held her off so I could nurse. 'I didn't dare give her a bottle,' he told me. He really understood how much I was going to need to nurse."

"My husband relieved my engorgement one night when we were away from the baby at an overnight party," recalls Sharon I. "We had never left the baby this long before, and by four in the morning I was so big—my breasts bulged and hurt. So I said to my husband, 'Hey, Mark's not here. Take over.' He drank all the milk and we went to sleep and everything was fine."

Although Sharon knows other couples who have used this method, she admits that this request will seem above and beyond the call of duty for many fathers and outlandish to others. In fact, her husband "thought it a bit strange" at first. "He said it was awkward, that he felt like a little baby again. But I nursed for seventeen months, and during that time he was willing to do it once in a while because he knew he was helping me out and making me more comfortable."

Many women do report that their partners sample the milk, just to experience the taste. One father said, "I wanted to find out what all the fuss was about."

Whether or not you ever have a taste test is not nearly as important as how you perceive a woman's breasts. Because breasts are an integral part of sexual foreplay for many couples, it can be easy to confuse this role with the main purpose of the breasts—to suckle and nourish a baby. If you feel awkward or uncomfortable when your partner breastfeeds, your attitude can make her more anxious and possibly inhibit the let-down reflex—not to mention her emotional need to have your undivided support and the knowledge that you see breastfeeding as a beautiful act of love. When you think about it, that a woman's body is capable of producing all the food your newborn needs is truly awesome. Make sure you tell her how proud you feel.

As the partner of a working/breastfeeding woman, there will be a lot of slack for you to take up. What follows are ideas of where and when your help is not only appreciated but downright essential.

Understand breastfeeding, how milk is produced, the let-down reflex, and the balance of supply and demand. (See Chapters One through Four, and consult "Resources" at the end of this book.) Your partner needs lots of confidence, and she will turn to you more often than anyone else when she has questions or concerns. The more you know about breastfeeding, the more you can help her and your baby.

Help your partner eat a well-balanced diet. Good food is essential to her health and to the production of milk that is rich in nutrients. (See Chapter Three, page 47.) Share in shopping, meal planning, and cooking. Pack nutritional snacks for her to take to work, and pack her lunch if she is planning to express milk during her lunch break. Discourage her from dieting, and remind her (and yourself) that because breastfeeding uses extra calories, she will gradually and safely return to her prepregnancy size if she maintains a healthy, well-balanced diet.

Help in the saving and storing of breastmilk. Shop for the supplies she will need to express milk at work. (See Chapter Five.) Help her wash and prepare containers, label milk, pack her supplies. Buy her a new briefcase, a carry pack, a cooler, or a tote.

Help your baby adjust to feeding from a bottle. Sometimes breastfed babies resist taking milk from a bottle. They don't like the nipple. The suckling action is different from mother's breast. And it is not unusual for breastfed babies to refuse a bottle when it is offered by the mother. "Why can't I have the breast?" they think indignantly. The adjustment to the bottle goes more smoothly when prompted by someone other than the mother. When your partner begins planning her return to work and the time comes to introduce the bottle, you can take over this job. You can begin with breastmilk she has expressed and saved, or with formula. Most fathers are eager for their turn to feed the baby. Some begin by giving a bottle when mother is out of the house socializing or running errands. This gives her a nice break, too. (See Chapter Four, page 84, for more information about introducing the bottle.)

Give other nourishment to your baby. Your baby has lots of other needs besides nursing. Each contact you have with her—from changing to rocking to looking into each other's eyes—is a vital part of baby care. Make the most of these moments, and experience skin-to-skin contact whenever you can (hold her against your bare chest, take her in your bath).

Help your partner get enough rest. Fatigue is the worst enemy of all new mothers, and your partner will be particularly susceptible when she returns to work. Remind her to take short naps whenever she can, and assure her that you will take care of the baby and anything else that needs to be done.

Put a "sh-h-h-h, mother sleeping" note on the door, and keep company to a minimum during the early weeks. When guests come to see the baby, it may be up to you to run interference or shoo them away if you see that she is getting tired.

Ease up on yourselves. You will both need to relax your housekeeping standards. Decide together what absolutely has to be done, and let the rest slide until the baby is older and your routine is better established. Keep meals simple, and do the chores and housework anytime you can.

Help at the end of the day. Your partner will probably need to sit down and nurse as soon as she gets home from work. You can help by straightening up and getting dinner started.

Help with a fussy baby. Nearly all babies have a fussy period each day. We all get tired, and babies are no exception. Encourage your partner to take a short rest or a warm bath while you walk, rock, or soothe the baby.

Share in finding day care. The decision about your baby's day care should be one you make together, including the first interviews and visits to the caregiver's, the drop-off and pick-up, and the communication with the caregiver about concerns and problems. (See Chapter Five, page 103.)

Help during the workday. Your own work schedule may be flexible, allowing you to bring the baby to Mom's workplace for a lunchtime nursing. In any case, you can share in the morning and afternoon transportation to and from the caregiver's.

Talk about your feelings. Some men feel awkward or self-conscious about breastfeeding, particularly in public, or they are bothered by their partners' breastfeeding or expressing milk at the job site. It is very important for you both to talk about these feelings openly and honestly. Know and understand each other's preferences, and then work out an arrangement that puts you both at ease. Breastfeeding can be accomplished smoothly and discreetly with the help of front-buttoning blouses, shawls, sweaters, or simply a light blanket draped loosely over the baby's head. You can keep a newspaper handy, to open and read as your partner nurses behind it. In public or at social gatherings, help her find a separate room, a quiet corner, or some privacy in which to nurse. And if she is having trouble negotiating her workday arrangements, either because the logistics are difficult or because she has no support from her coworkers, she will need extra encouragement and constructive suggestions from you.

Be patient with your sex life. Many couples (whether breast- or bottle-feeding) experience a period of sexual adjustment after the birth of a baby. Sometimes women are nervous about resuming intercourse. Talking about these feelings, along with a gentle, unhurried approach, will help the two of you get started again. A number of breastfeeding women report that their desire for sex wanes while they are nursing. (See the following chapter: "Sex and the Breastfeeding Woman.")

Share responsibility for birth control. A woman is less likely to conceive while breastfeeding because she has high levels of the hormone prolactin, which inhibits ovulation. However, it *is* still possible to become pregnant during this time. The amount of protection breastfeeding provides depends on whether the baby is breastfed exclusively (no supplements), the length of time between feedings, and whether the baby is allowed to nurse for comfort between feedings. Discuss contraception with your practitioner before you resume intercourse. Foam, condoms, and diaphragms are okay to use while breastfeeding. Current research has raised some question as to the safety of IUDs (intrauterine devices). The pill and minipill are not recommended while breastfeeding because of the unknown effects the added hormones can have on the baby. (For more information, see "Contraceptives," page 169.)

Good Gifts for a Working/Breastfeeding Mom

In case anyone asks, don't hesitate to mention what your partner *really* needs. How about . . .?

- Dinner sent in from your favorite restaurant.
- Housekeeping or cleaning services for a day, a week, or longer (if your giver is especially generous).
- Babysitting so you two can go out together.
- A dinner or casserole (the best are those that can be refrigerated or frozen and heated when you most need them).
- An invitation to Sunday brunch.
- A basket of fresh fruit.
- Taxi service to and from the caregiver's for the noon feeding.
- A gift certificate for laundry service.
- Child care or caregiver's fees for a week.
- A new briefcase, tote, or carry pack for her breastfeeding supplies.
- Groceries delivered to your home.
- Coming over on Saturday to do the yard work.
- Doing a basket of your ironing.
- A gift certificate for a hair cut, wash and set, or perm.
- A gift certificate for a massage, facial, or manicure.
- Diaper service for a week, a month, or longer.
- Nursing clothes, either purchased or hand made.

❧ 10

Sex and the Breastfeeding Woman

What sex life?" was one new mother's response when we asked how hers was going.

"Who cares?" another said, adding that she lost interest in sex during the time she was breastfeeding. And that caused a problem with her husband. "He didn't appreciate it, and thought it was because I was breastfeeding."

Lillian N. mentioned problems with vaginal lubrication (not enough) and disconcerting milk let-down during intercourse. "I leaked all over the place when we made love," she says. Kim C. recalls that it "took forever to get aroused—I didn't have an orgasm for a year."

Margaret L., who worked and breastfed two children, had the same experience. "I don't like sex at all when I'm breastfeeding. But I feel guilty all the time. When we do have sex, I just want to get it over with, and I'm glad because I don't have to feel guilty again for a couple of days.

"I don't know if it's breastfeeding, or because I have a new baby and I'm tired. I'm always so glad I can finally get to sleep that I just don't want to think about having to do anything else. I often thought if I could just stop worrying about getting enough sleep, maybe I could relax and enjoy this. But when you have two kids and are breastfeeding, and you're into the kids all day, all you want to do when they're finally in bed is to go to sleep."

Margaret's husband, however, did some reading and was glad to find out that this has happened to other new mothers. As a result, he is understanding and patient. Other fathers, though, blame breastfeeding for their wives' waning amorous advances, and this can generate conflict and misunderstanding. In some instances, this reaction stems from a type of sexual jealousy of the breastfed infant, particularly if the baby is a male and is older than six months. Often fathers push for weaning because they simply want their wives back.

A great number of women lose interest in sex when they are breastfeeding, even though there is little scientific evidence to show whether lactation is or is not the culprit. However, lower sex drive is associated with the postpartum period, because women who have just given birth often experience a temporary decrease in the level of estrogen hormone. Low estrogen can also cause less vaginal lubrication, which makes intercourse more difficult and sometimes painful.

It is possible that breastfeeding mothers experience a decreased sex drive longer than non-breastfeeding mothers, though there is no scientific data to support such a conclusion. In fact, one Masters and Johnson study (cited by Ruth A. Lawrence in *Breastfeeding: A Guide for the Medical Profession*) found that nursing mothers were more anxious to resume sex than non-nursing mothers. Dr. Lawrence also observes that while some women have an increased interest in sex, others have no interest at all for up to six months after birth.

Dr. Lawrence does not draw any definitive conclusions to explain the loss of sex drive, but she does suggest these possibilities: 1. Nursing fulfills the mother's needs for intimacy and stimulus; 2. The let-down reflex and milk ejection sometimes triggered by sexual arousal is a turnoff for some men; 3. Many women are fatigued; 4. Many women fear pregnancy.

Fatigue is a reality among new mothers, especially when they return to work. Also, the adjustment to being parents and the constant demands of a new baby can wreak havoc on marital relationships. And until the baby begins to sleep through the night, the expectation of interruptions can interfere with sexual pleasure. Suddenly the night belongs to the baby. And for both parents, it's easy to get wrapped up in the baby and forget to take time out for each other.

Knowing that these problems are shared by other new parents is probably the best way to understand and accept what is happening to you. Patience is essential. Time is on your side. Get as much rest as you can. Before long the baby will be sleeping through the night, will be breastfeeding less, and you will fall into a more manageable routine.

In the meantime, it is important for the two of you to talk about your feelings. Find some time for each other, even if you have to make an appointment. Pick a time when the baby will be sleeping, and promise to spend that time together rather than catching up on housework. Breastfeed before sex, to lower the amount of milk in the breast and to help assure that the baby will stay asleep. Hire someone you trust to take care of the baby, and have a special night out each week. As for sex, select times when you can both relax and enjoy each other. (Okay, maybe it won't be as spontaneous as it used to be.)

On the weekends, try afternoon naps or showers together while the baby is sleeping. Or rent a motel room for the night and leave the baby with a caregiver you trust. Light some candles near the bed. Arrange an afternoon off together, but pick up the baby at the usual time.

Talk about your sexual relationship and be honest about what works and does not work, what you like and don't like. For example, some women find a side-to-side position more comfortable because there is less pressure on the vaginal area that may still be tender from an episiotomy. Couples who have never used vaginal lubrication often find they need it during this period.

Remember that other types of physical contact can be satisfying expressions of love—holding each other, massage and back rubs, and cuddling—until you get your sexual relationship started again.

BREASTS AND SEX

The breasts respond to all phases of a woman's sexuality (menstruation, sexual intercourse, pregnancy, childbirth, and lactation), most noticeably through enlargement and/or nipple changes. This is because the hormonal interactions in all these events of a woman's cycle are similar.

Thus, some women experience a form of sexual gratification during suckling on certain occasions, and the handling and manipulation of the breasts during lactation can be stimulating in some circumstances. However, the majority of women who enjoy breastfeeding and who find the intimacy with their infants pleasant and satisfying are *not* having a response we would label as sexual arousal.

The breasts are designed for nurturing and nourishing an infant, and nursing and suckling are natural, biological phenomena. If this function is confused with the breasts' reputation and secondary role as objects of sexual interest, feelings of anxiety and embarrassment can result. As a working/breastfeeding mother, you may find yourself in settings characterized by just such ambivalence toward breasts. Many men (and some women) are uncomfortable with or offended by breastfeeding. If you are confident and at ease with what you are doing, you will be less troubled by these attitudes and may help to change them. In any event, you will want to approach nonsupportive situations one step at a time. As one woman put it: "It's fine to think we could sit at our desks and pump milk, but frankly, it's going to be a long time before that happens."

CONTRACEPTIVES

Lactation will protect against pregnancy to some degree, but it is not foolproof. Whether or not you can become pregnant while you are breastfeeding will depend on several factors, among them how often you nurse and whether the baby receives any supplemental feedings. If you want to be absolutely sure you don't conceive, it is wise to consult your physician about your birth control options. Don't wait until you begin menstruating to start using birth control. Ovulation can occur before your first postpartum menstrual period.

Diaphragms, condoms, vaginal creams, suppositories, and jellies are not associated with any harmful effects during breastfeeding. In the past there has been concern in the medical community about the use of IUD's (intrauterine devices). Studies have linked IUD's with heavy bleeding, pelvic infections, and tube damage. Whether breastfeeding or not, you should discuss thoroughly your contraceptive options with your physician before making a choice. For a useful pamphlet entitled *Contraception*, send a stamped, self-addressed business-size envelope to the American College of Obstetricians and Gynecologists, Resource Center, 409 12th Street SW, P.O. Box 96920, Washington, D.C. 20090-6920.

Your (Legal) Right to Breastfeed

Before her first baby was born, Judy Deeley prepared to the hilt. She attended classes on lactating. Knowing she wanted to continue breastfeeding after she returned to work from maternity leave, she carefully outlined a plan, and wrote to her employer, the Clerk of Court for Pinellas County, Florida. She asked simply for flexible break times, so that she could pump her milk, and for a place in which to pump.

When her employer failed to answer her request, Judy returned to work and pumped her milk in an empty office on her break. Two days later, she received notification that her request was denied, and her employer suggested Judy wean the baby. Further, Judy was told not to use any room in the building to pump and not to use the refrigerators to store milk, or the facilities to wash the equipment. She was told that someone had raised concerns about the transmission of the virus that causes AIDS. Judy was offered a job located closer to home, in a position that was a demotion.

Forbidden to use the building, Judy went outside into her car and pumped her milk with a battery pump. After that, she was formally reprimanded for insubordination. However, the press got hold of the story, and a news broadcast of Judy in her car in the intense Florida noontime heat caught the attention of a local attorney, Patricia Lee. Lee specializes in family law and has a special interest in breastfeeding laws and litigation. Lee helped Judy file her grievance with the company. A hearing was held in which Lee argued the benefits of breastfeeding to the baby, the benefits to the company when employees' needs are accommodated, and breastfeeding as a right protected by the U.S. Constitution. The process was emotionally grueling, but the result was that the county government removed the reprimands from Deeley's file and allowed her the flexible scheduling she needed to pump milk. Later, the county government adopted a policy in support of breastfeeding mothers, granted flex time to accommodate pumping, and agreed to provide, where possible, a clean and private area for pumping and provisions for storage of milk. The year was 1994.

Deeley continued to work and breastfeed, although she never was given a private room in which to pump. Of this partial victory, Lee said, "We couldn't get her out of the bathroom, but we got her flex time, and she was allowed to do it. Although it felt like a big coup and a great success, [Judy] was saddened by the reaction. She just wanted to take care of her baby."

A PLACE FOR BREASTFEEDING IN YOUR PLACE OF WORK

When breastfeeding a baby and working become difficult or impossible to combine, we automatically assume that breastfeeding is the obstacle underlying all the complications. In fact, this whole book has been based on the reality that breastfeeding and working is one of the trickiest of all the juggling acts women perform in order to be employed outside the home. To breastfeed while working, women need determination, creativity, support, and lots of strategies and accoutrements. When something has to give, it is usually the breastfeeding, not the job, that is abandoned. Employer policies or attitudes in the workplace that have either tacitly or openly sabotaged the breastfeeding effort are not usually changed.

The purpose of this chapter is certainly not to diminish the material that has been presented but rather to look at the working/breastfeeding issue from a slightly different perspective. For a moment, let's ask the question that has been hovering in the wings throughout this entire book: *Why* is breastfeeding and working such a difficult combination?

Certainly, when you inject another responsibility or activity into your working life there are adjustments to be made and extra pressures to cope with. However, to assume there is something inherently incompatible in being a parent and having a job is to ignore both our own potential and the ability of the workplace to adapt to the dramatic changes in families' and particularly women's lives. The issue here is not just breastfeeding mothers; it is working mothers. The "balancing act" we all must perform in order to participate and compete in the workplace is more than finding a private room in which to pump milk discreetly. True, this can be one of the most important daily concerns, but it is only the tip of the iceberg. What lies below is the fact that the American workplace, for the most part, is not set up to accommodate the nurturing of children. We have learned to accept that when compromises must be made, it is the parenting side of our lives that has to give.

Traditionally, the workplace has segregated our personal from our professional lives. We go to work and quickly learn that it is not appropriate to bring along our concerns about family and children. Really successful people might bring the office home, but they never bring the home into the office. While our purpose here is not to track this attitude historically, it seems obvious that the domination of the workforce by men could be cited as having significant influence here: As long as women were at home taking care of the children, it was possible for men to go to work and leave their toddlers' troubles behind. It was also possible to structure the workplace as a setting where things having to do with babies and kids simply don't belong. And the economy hums along with the worker bees at work and the primary caregiver bees at home.

Now what happens when women enter the work force? We know what happens in our households—everything goes topsy-turvy as roles are reversed, redefined, and shuffled. And it isn't just the working mother who has brought about this change in family structure. Fathers are opting for more involvement in parenting. They don't want to be bystanders; they want to be nurturers as well, and they are increasingly rejecting the claims their jobs have made against their time as fathers. Many parents are now questioning the long-held belief that working and parenting must imply a choice between two mismatched roles.

Your desire to be a working/breastfeeding mother is the epitomal challenge to the assumption that working and parenting are mutually exclusive. You are not just bringing parenting into the workplace because you are a mother; you are bringing in specific and visible mothering functions. You have a breast pump in your drawer. You carry bottles of breastmilk around in a cooler. Perhaps your baby is brought to you during your lunch hour. You have large breasts that sometimes leak milk. The obvious fact you are nursing a baby is not easily left behind at home. *Nor should it be.*

Remember the puzzles in children's activity books that show an illustration captioned "What's wrong with this picture?" In the case of the working mother's scenario, a lot is wrong. We have been led to believe that in order to have satisfying or successful careers, we must "fit" mothering into our work lives. The workplace says to us: Look, it's great to have babies, as long as they are out of the picture at work. Matters pertaining to children do not belong here. Keep that stuff under wraps. As for breastfeeding, this is totally inappropriate.

What's wrong with this picture? It's that the very nature of the workplace excludes persons who are caring for children. But remember, the workplace was originally designed with men's, not women's, needs in mind. As long as the structure of the workplace stays the same, those people who need to both work and nurture children will be successful only insofar as they can balance and juggle against the odds. This is particularly true with regard to breastfeeding. The acceptance and support the workplace gives to nursing women will be a measure of how skillful and discreet breastfeeding women can be. The less intrusive your breastfeeding, the more positive will be the response to what you're doing. See the irony? We will "make strides" by demonstrating how well we can accommodate our parenting to our working lives. The balancing act is women and men *acting* like they are not mothers and fathers, and thus keeping the workplace in *balance.*

The United States lags behind the growing number of countries that have national policies supporting the presence of breastfeeding women in the workplace. Even maternity leaves, though guaranteed in some states under certain circumstances, are not uniform throughout the country, and in many cases must be negotiated. The maternity leave concept itself applies to the needs of the mother, but policies do not extend to include the child or breastfeeding, which is a need of the child. When maternity leave is granted as a right under the Pregnancy Discrimination Act (to be discussed in detail later), again the concern is the mother's ability to return to work. There are no provisions in this Act to include the method of feeding the child as a reason to extend the leave. And while many companies are providing child care facilities in response to the burgeoning number of women in the work force, cost is high and capacity is low, and the demand still far outdistances the supply. As far as flex-time, paternity leaves, and sick leaves when children are ill are concerned, the trend is slow.

As a working/breastfeeding woman, you probably already know that you are pioneering through some new territory. How difficult it has been for you to blaze your path depends to a great extent on your work environment. If you work in a totally supportive setting, where you are able to breastfeed or express milk easily at work and remain flexible to the needs of your child, you are fortunate, and your place of employment already has the components of an ideal. Or maybe you have been able to pull off working and breastfeeding without upsetting anyone's apple cart—by keeping a low profile and simply avoiding the issue. In this case, you have made a lot of compromises for the sake of your baby, and you probably wish it could have been easier. If, on the other hand, your job has made breastfeeding difficult or impossible, and your mothering and your job are locked in an either/or conflict, something has to change.

That something does not necessarily have to be your breastfeeding. In fact, you have a right to expect support from the workplace for the kind of parenting you choose. And the larger the number of women who approach jobs with this attitude, the sooner the overall consciousness will rise to meet them.

At this point there is no clear mandate for employers to permit female employees to breastfeed on the premises, nor do they have to give consideration to extending or flexing breaks for feeding a baby or expressing milk, or to flexing work schedules to accommodate child care. Those women who face recalcitrant employers are breaking new ground, and there is not a huge pile of jurisprudence to support the cause. Cases in which women have sought legal recourse for the right to breastfeed are few and far between.

In "When Private Goes Public: Legal Protection for Women Who Breastfeed in Public and at Work" (*Law and Inequality: A Journal of Theory and Practice,* December 1995), author Danielle M. Shelton writes: "Until a clear and feasible policy protecting breastfeeding and breastpumping is established, many women may be forced to choose unnecessarily between their jobs, their public lives, and the well-being of their children."

In the following pages we will discuss three key lawsuits brought by women who were denied the right to work and breastfeed: 1. *Board of School Directors of Fox Chapel Area School District v. Cheryl Y. Rossetti;* 2. *Janice Davis Dike v. School Board of Orange County, Florida;* 3. *Linda Eaton v. City of Iowa and City of Iowa Fire Department.* Besides being interesting, these cases are very important because they form the beginnings of the framework for interpretation of the law as it applies to the working/breastfeeding issue. If you are being discriminated against in your efforts to work and breastfeed your baby, these cases have aspects that may help you and your legal advisor(s) build your own case.

We will tell the stories of these three women in chronological order. However, the most notable suit as far as establishing a useful legal precedent is *Dike v. School Board of Orange County, Florida.* This particular case is a landmark because it clearly establishes that breastfeeding is *protected* by the Constitution.

In "A Guide to Your Legal Rights," we'll talk about state and federal laws that protect breastfeeding mothers. The next section, "Negotiate First," gives suggestions for coming to an agreement with your employer without resorting to legal redress, and the final sections give you guidelines for filing a lawsuit, finding an attorney, and garnering support for your cause.

BREASTFEEDING GOES TO COURT: THREE CASES

Please keep in mind as you read these cases that the chances are probably slim that it will be necessary for you to carry your working/breastfeeding choice into the courtroom, or even to a lawyer's office. Should you ever need it, however, this material can serve as a resource, giving you a realistic picture of your rights as a parent and of the legal precedents and parameters that have been established in this area.

Board of School Directors of Fox Chapel v. Rossetti 387 A. 2nd 957 (Cmwlth. Ct. Pa., 1978)

(This case was an appeal brought by the school board in an effort to reverse a decision by the secretary of education to reinstate Cheryl Y. Rossetti after she had been fired from her teaching position in the Fox Chapel area school district.)

On October 18, 1975, Cheryl Rossetti, an elementary teacher, gave birth to a son. In her contract, she was allowed an eight-week maternity leave, which could be extended at thirty-day intervals if she provided the school district with a physician's certificate that the extension was necessary for her recovery.

In December, shortly before she was scheduled to return to work, Rossetti presented a letter from her obstetrician and was granted a four-week extension of her leave. Then, in January, before these four weeks were over, Rossetti sent a letter to the district superintendent requesting leave for the rest of the school year so that she could breastfeed her child.

In summary, her reasons were twofold: First, Rossetti suffered from allergies so serious that she received weekly injections. She hoped that breastfeeding her son would help reduce his chances of inheriting her allergy problems, and, in fact, a pediatrician testified to this likelihood at a later hearing. Second, her son refused to drink from a bottle, even when the bottle contained her breastmilk. Short of a stomach tube, breastfeeding was the only way for Cheryl Rossetti to feed her son. At this time, he was breastfeeding on demand five to seven times a day.

The superintendent's reply to Rossetti's letter stated that there were no provisions in her contract to grant any further leave. At this point, Rossetti appeared at the school board meeting, with a representative of the Pennsylvania State Education Association, to request that she be granted a discretionary leave (as opposed to a maternity leave). The board denied the request, and Rossetti was told to report to work the next day.

She didn't. Instead, she wrote another letter to the superintendent explaining that her son's need to breastfeed made it impossible for her to return to work as requested. Also, her union representative wrote a letter to the superintendent on her behalf. On January 29, a special board meeting was held, and the superintendent drew up a list of charges against Rossetti. She was charged with violating a section of the public school code through "persistent negligence . . . persistent or willful violation of the school laws of this Commonwealth . . . [and] incompetency." Again Rossetti argued the reasons she needed to breastfeed her son. The board voted to deny her request. However, the secretary later reversed the denial and ordered that Rossetti be reinstated. The board appealed. On June 13, 1978, the judge of the Commonwealth Court of Pennsylvania upheld the secretary's decision.

In the opinion, Judge DiSalle did not agree with the charges that Cheryl Rossetti was persistently negligent, that she willfully violated the school's laws, or that she was incompetent, stating that while these charges are valid reasons for termination, "(Rossetti's) conduct cannot be characterized as rising to this level." The judge stated that she was conscientious in her efforts to inform the board and to obtain its approval for her actions, and that considering the circumstances, she felt she had no choice but to continue to stay home after the board ordered her to return to work. The judge also said that her decision not to return to work was "reasonable," since "no other person was capable of performing the maternal duties required of her."

Rossetti had argued that to deny her further leave of absence to breastfeed her child constituted a pregnancy-based discrimination in violation of the Pennsylvania Human Relations Act. Previous case law in that state interpreted pregnancy-based discrimination as sex-based discrimination, since only women can bear children. In one case cited in the Rossetti opinion, a judge had stated that since pregnancy is unique to women, any disability plan that denies benefits for pregnancy also discriminates against women because of their sex.

The judge in the Rossetti case extended this interpretation to include breastfeeding, since breastfeeding is also something only women can do. The judge stated: ". . . since the development of the law in this area has been based upon the unique position of the female confronted with the prospect of childbirth, it follows that the request for additional leave for breastfeeding purposes . . . is merely a logical and natural extension of that concept." The judge stated that the refusal of the school board to grant Rossetti an unpaid leave for breastfeeding amounted to unlawful discrimination under the state's Human Relations Act.

This case used sex discrimination as the basis for a breastfeeding lawsuit, raising civil rights issues, and suggested that Title VII and the Pregnancy Discrimination Act (described later) might be interpreted to include protection for women who feel they are being discriminated against in their choice to breastfeed. However, it is important to know that at this stage there are no antidiscrimination laws that apply to child rearing—only to disability resulting from pregnancy and birth. Thus, a case brought on the basis of discrimination will require an interpretation of existing laws to include breastfeeding.

Janice Davis Dike v. School Board of Orange County, Florida 650 F. 2nd 783 (5th Cir., 1981)

Janice Dike is an elementary teacher who arranged to breastfeed her baby during her duty-free lunch break at school. Her husband brought the baby to school at about 11:30 A.M., and Dike breastfed in the privacy of a locked room. If she was needed by the school during this hour, her husband would take the baby while she performed her duties.

Janice Dike breastfed on this routine for three months. Then, when the school principal finally got wind of it, he told her to stop. His reason was that the school board rules prohibited teachers from bringing their children to work with them. He told Dike that she would be disciplined if she continued to breastfeed at school.

Dike complied. She stopped breastfeeding at noon, and her baby was supplemented with formula. However, the baby developed a formula allergy. At this point Dike expressed milk to be given at the noon feeding, but the baby showed signs of being emotionally upset, and Dike's concern affected her own well-being. She then asked if she could either leave the school at noon to go home and breastfeed or breastfeed the baby in her camper van in the parking lot. Both requests were denied. This time the school board said they had another policy prohibiting teachers from leaving school premises during the day.

When her baby began refusing the bottle altogether, Janice Dike had no choice but to take an unpaid leave for the rest of the school year. She sued the school board, charging that it had interfered with her constitutional right to nurture her child by breastfeeding.

The district court barely gave Dike the time of day. Her case was quickly dismissed on the grounds that it was "frivolous" (which means it is a waste of the court's time), and the judge said it was okay for the school board to prohibit breastfeeding on school grounds. Dike, represented by the attorneys for the Florida Teaching Profession—National Education Association, appealed the case to the U.S. Circuit Court of Appeals. Here, Dike's claim was accepted as having merit, and the judge ordered the district court to give her a trial.

Two issues were defined in Dike's case. First, the judge of the Court of Appeals stated that Dike's interest in breastfeeding was entitled to constitutional protection. On the other hand, he also recognized that the school board might have legitimate reasons for policies that prevent the disruption of the school day (such as teachers bringing children to school). However, he said that her claim should not have been dismissed by the lower court and that she was entitled to a trial.

Dike's case rested on constitutional law, and specifically on the Ninth and Fourteenth Amendments. The judicial opinion is very significant because it establishes constitutional protection for breastfeeding on the grounds that breastfeeding is a "fundamental right." When a fundamental right is established, the state must have "compelling reasons" to interfere with that right.

The judge of the Court of Appeals, who authored the opinion, stated in his analysis that "the Constitution protects from undue state interference citizens' freedom of personal choice in some areas of marriage and family life." Protected liberties include decisions affecting marriage, procreation, contraception, abortion, and family relationships. Further, he cited the Supreme Court's long-held recognition that "parents' interest in nurturing and rearing their children deserves special protection against state interference."

"Breastfeeding is the most elemental form of parental care," he goes on. "It is communion between mother and child that, like marriage, is 'intimate to the degree of being sacred' [from *Griswold v. Connecticut*]." He concluded that "the Constitution protects from excessive state interference a woman's decision respecting breastfeeding her child." But the Judge pointed out that this did not mean that the school board's restriction necessarily had violated the Constitution. Whether or not the regulations were too rigid was a matter to be determined at trial.

Back to the district court. The trial was held, but this judge (the same one who dismissed the case the first time) ruled in favor of the school board, saying that it had the right to prohibit breastfeeding. This ruling of the lower court is interesting and a bit disturbing. Usually when a fundamental right is established, as it was by the judge of the Court of Appeals, it is unusual for this right to be overruled. As mentioned before, the state must have compelling—very strong—reasons to interfere with this right. Thus, by ruling as it did, the lower (district) court said that the school's policy of not allowing teachers' children on the school grounds was compelling; that is, it was so important to the interests of education that it justified interfering with an individual's fundamental right.

Whether or not the school's interest was compelling is certainly open to debate. While the necessity of the policy regarding children might be sensible and rational, it may not be "compelling." From a legal standpoint, there is a big difference.

Dike and her attorneys headed back to the U.S. Circuit Court of Appeals. In the meantime, however, the school board decided to propose a settlement out of court. The board had already spent a great deal of money and had endured a lot of public embarrassment for its stance in this case. Dike accepted the settlement. She received back pay and was reinstated in her job. It took three years for the case to be resolved.

What makes the Dike case landmark is that it established breastfeeding as a right under the Ninth and Fourteenth Amendments of the Constitution. Ideally, for a state to encroach on this right, it must have very compelling reasons. It should be stressed that the fact that the lower court opinion in this case found that the school had a compelling interest that overruled Dike's fundamental right is not particularly good news for the breastfeeding issue. However, the school board's decision to propose a settlement before the case got back to the Court of Appeals is probably an indication of its expectation that the Court of Appeals would reverse the decision and rule in favor of Dike's fundamental right.

When a woman argues a case based on *Dike*, Danielle Shelton suggests that she stress the sincerity of her belief that breastfeeding is best for her baby, bring studies that show the unarguable health benefits of breastfeeding, and emphasize her belief that breastfeeding is an integral part of parenting, not merely a personal preference.

[In both the Rossetti and Dike cases, the baby was allergic to formula and thus breastfeeding was essential. However, the Dike case in particular did not rest on the baby's allergies, but rather on the parent's fundamental right to breastfeed. We must not assume that we have to have an "excuse"—such as an allergic child—to justify the desire to breastfeed. Breastfeeding is justified regardless of whether a formula alternative is possible.]

Linda Eaton v. City of Iowa City and City of Iowa City Fire Department

Most people remember her as "the firefighter in Iowa," and to others she is a legend. Linda Eaton's battle over the right to breastfeed her child in the fire station is the most pub-

licized breastfeeding case on record. Within a few days after
the press got word of the case, over eighty media sources—fifteen overseas—had contacted Eaton's attorney. *The New York
Times* followed the story throughout, and features appeared in
Ms. magazine.

This case struck a cord, and people were fascinated by
this woman's chutzpah. Not only did Linda Eaton challenge
the most exclusive of all male bastions—the firehouse—but
she did it with the most womanly of all womanly functions—
breastfeeding. As it turned out, the institution couldn't handle
such a multitiered affront.

It started in January 1979, when Linda Eaton returned
from maternity leave to her job as a firefighter with the Iowa
City Fire Department. She asked the chief if she could have
her son brought to the station for two breastfeedings each
day. The plan was to breastfeed her son during her personal
time (time allotted firefighters for eating, sleeping, playing
cards, showering, etc.) in the women's locker area. The baby
would be brought to the station by Eaton's mother.

The chief denied the request, citing a rule (it was later
learned that this rule was "unwritten") that forbade visitors on
the premises during a firefighter's duty shift. On her first day
back on the job, Eaton had the baby brought to the station as
planned. She was suspended for the day and was told that she
would receive further disciplinary action, including dismissal,
if she did not comply with the chief's denial of her request.
On her next duty shift, she again had the baby brought to the
station and was again suspended for the remainder of that
day's shift.

Eaton filed for an injunction in the Johnson County district court, which would stop the city from punishing her. As
a result, a temporary restraining order was issued, allowing her
to return to her job and barring the city from taking any puni-
tive action against her until a trial could be held.

This strategy was devised by Eaton's attorney, Clara Ole-
son, specifically for the purpose of buying time so that her
client could continue to breastfeed and also be spared the ex-

treme pressure of a lawsuit during the time she was lactating. The complaint was first filed in the district court, asking for temporary injunctive relief. Then the civil rights suit was filed with the request that the injunction be kept in effect until the case was litigated. Since it took months before the case was heard by the Civil Rights Commission, Eaton was able to stay on the job and continue breastfeeding while the case was being prepared.

The city did propose conciliation. Eaton was offered alternative positions as a bus driver, a maintenance worker, an animal control officer, and a police dispatcher. Understandably, she responded that these were unacceptable options to firefighting.

In March of that year, the case was sent to the Iowa Civil Rights Commission for a hearing. Specifically, the complaint was filed under a state statute, alleging that Linda Eaton's right to privacy was violated. The commission unanimously ruled that Linda Eaton had been discriminated against, and she was awarded $2,000 in compensatory payment and $145.12 in back pay, and her attorneys were awarded $26,000 for their fees. In the opinion of the commission, the city had used an "obscure rule" (that visitors are not allowed in the firehouse) to institute a no-nursing policy that denied Eaton her civil rights.

When her son was seventeen months old, Eaton was still nursing him at the firehouse. Sounds like a happy and just ending to the story? Not exactly. She may have had legal backing, but she had little support from her coworkers or from the city. Linda Eaton was the brunt of firehouse pranks, jokes, hostility, and verbal abuse. She found salt in her orange juice; her photograph was blackened. In the written decision of the Iowa Civil Rights Commission (April 17, 1980), "retaliatory acts and harassment" against Eaton were charged to have begun as soon as she initiated the district court proceedings. The Commission stated: "She suffered an increased number of reprimands, a radical change in the nature of evaluations, the creation of a special visitors' log [Eaton's nursings were recorded in a separate log from that of the personal visitors other firefighters entertained while on duty]."

The city refused to take action, and the harassment continued. In fact, on May 1, 1980, the city council voted to appeal the decision of the Iowa Civil Rights Commission. Finally, on May 15, 1980, Linda Eaton resigned. Earlier that day, while responding to a fire, she found that the middle fingers of her work gloves had been cut off. Now the pranks were becoming life threatening. Later she was quoted in *The New York Times* as saying: "It just got subtly unbearable."

Linda Eaton brought a sexual harassment suit against the city, charging that the firefighters harassed her and that the city did nothing to help. She claimed $940,000 in damages and $324,000 in lost earnings and back pay. In February 1984, the three-week-long trial was held in Iowa City. The jury ruled against Eaton, stating that "horseplay and rough language" are a part of life in the firehouse. But what isn't a part of life in the firehouse, it would appear, is breastfeeding. At least not in Iowa City.

Remember, however, that Linda Eaton did receive a favorable decision from the Iowa Civil Rights Commission regarding her desire to breastfeed. This is a positive legal precedent. In every respect, Linda Eaton took the system to task. First she stepped into a profession that has been tenaciously guarded by and for men, then she showed with great determination how mothering and firefighting could be combined. She was willing to take her commitment to breastfeeding to court and weathered what everyone who files discrimination fears: retaliation. This is the kind of front-line courage that will open doors for all of us.

To *The New York Times,* she said: "If any nursing mother can use me for any kind of example of inspiration, then it's well worth it, because it's the best way to start out a baby, I think."

A GUIDE TO YOUR LEGAL RIGHTS

Currently, a number of states have or are considering legislation to protect breastfeeding women, including New York, Florida, Missouri, California, North Carolina, Tennessee, Illinois, Michigan, Utah, Virginia, Arizona, Ohio, Wisconsin, Texas, and Nevada. These laws range from protecting a woman from being arrested for indecency to exempting her from jury duty. The most pioneering laws are in Florida and New York. To date, New York is the only state to classify breastfeeding as a civil right. Florida's law (Florida Statutes Section 383.015), passed in 1993, is a public health law that states "A mother may breast feed her baby in any location, public or private, where the mother is otherwise authorized to be, irrespective of whether the nipple of the mother's breast is uncovered during or incidental to the breast feeding." In 1994, Florida passed supplementary legislation to create "baby-friendly" workplaces, beginning with a pilot project for state employees with worksite breastfeeding support, such as flexible scheduling and private space to pump. The Texas legislature passed similar provisions in 1995, adding to theirs a statement urging private businesses to accommodate breastfeeding mothers.

Most state laws do not specifically address breastfeeding in the workplace, but laws such as Florida's, which allow a woman to breastfeed anywhere it is legal for her to be, logically include the workplace. However, as far as litigation is concerned, these state laws have not yet impacted labor law disputes. New York's law is the only one that gives a woman legal remedy; in other words, she can bring a lawsuit against someone who has interfered with her right to breastfeed. Florida's law, on the other hand, offers women no legal recourse against those who discriminate against them.

Of the federal laws prohibiting discrimination against women workers, the one most pertinent to breastfeeding and parenting issues is: Title VII of the Civil Rights Act of 1964, amended by the Equal Employment Opportunity Act of 1972 and the Pregnancy Discrimination Act of 1978.

Title VII of the Civil Rights Act of 1964

This federal law prohibits employment discrimination on the basis of race, color, religion, sex, or national origin. Under Title VII, employment discrimination by any groups having fifteen or more employees is forbidden, including private employers, state and local governments, educational institutions, and labor organizations. In addition, the federal government, employment agencies, and joint labor-management committees for apprenticeship and training are regulated under this Act.

Title VII is very broad and comprehensive, and makes illegal nearly all situations where: 1. Hiring or employment policies treat women differently from men on the basis of their sex; 2. Policies have a disproportionately adverse effect on women (such as height and weight requirements); 3. An employer's official policies do not discriminate but the employer does, in fact, treat women differently. The last category is called disparate-treatment and is the legal framework most closely related to the breastfeeding issue. It is also, unfortunately, one of the hardest discrimination cases to win.

One way to look at disparate-treatment as it might apply to breastfeeding is this: Let's say that the terms of employment are not discriminatory; that is, they do not treat women any differently from men. However, when you try to devise a strategy for working and breastfeeding your baby, the structure of the job or the policies of the workplace make it impossible for you to do this (for example, work breaks are so rigidly structured that you cannot leave your assignment to pump milk, or, as in the Dike case, school board rules prohibited teachers' children being brought to the school grounds). In these situations, the terms of employment are not discriminatory in and of themselves, but they make it impossible for you to breastfeed without the risk of losing your job or being penalized in your chances for advancement.

This is where things get tricky. With no laws specifically protecting breastfeeding women, it becomes a matter of interpreting whether the employment policies discriminate in your particular case, and the extent to which Title VII protects you. It seems logical that if employment policies prevent women from parenting in the way they choose (i.e., through breastfeeding), and women are the only ones who can breastfeed, then sabotage of the breastfeeding effort is discriminatory. To take this line of reasoning a step further, if the workplace does not accommodate the care of children (within reason), and during breastfeeding the woman is clearly the primary caregiver, then the workplace is, in effect, excluding primary caregivers from equal opportunity and thus could be construed as discriminatory. In other words, *women cannot compete on equal footing with men in the workplace until their unique role as nurturers of children is taken into account.*

Here it is easy to make the error of thinking that we women are asking for "special treatment." That is because breastfeeding women cannot always fit into the employer's terms, even when those terms are not flagrantly discriminatory. The reason for this is that the system itself is not set up to accommodate the nurturing of children, especially with regard to breastfeeding. In order for breastfeeding to become a solidly and legally grounded right, women must continue to come forward and challenge the system's rigidity, and thus continue to chip away at the attitudes that have kept the doors of the workplace shut for so long.

The problem of what to do about functions that are unique to women was addressed and clarified by the Pregnancy Discrimination Act, and it is probably under the umbrella of this law that the breastfeeding issue falls.

The Pregnancy Discrimination Act of 1978

Signed into law by former President Jimmy Carter as an amendment to Title VII, the Pregnancy Discrimination Act (PDA) specifically forbids discrimination on the basis of pregnancy, childbirth, and related medical conditions. The PDA does not state that pregnancy is unique and thus requires special treatment. Rather, it places pregnancy (and related conditions) in the same basket with other disabilities that might affect a person's ability to do her/his job, or that would require a leave. Thus, pregnancy leave and disability policies must treat women under the same terms that are applied to other disabilities. For example, if jobs are held open for other disabled employees, then the jobs of pregnant or childbearing women must be held open on the same basis. Insurance and benefit policies must be the same for pregnancy as for other disabilities. Seniority policies must be the same for employees absent because of pregnancy as for those absent for other medical reasons.

The PDA establishes that discrimination against pregnant women is sex discrimination. Key here, then, is whether or not breastfeeding is a natural extension of pregnancy, and thus a "related medical condition" covered by the PDA. So far, no case has directly determined this. However, Shelton points out how breastfeeding and pregnancy are alike: "Both are quasi-voluntary conditions. Both are exclusively linked to women's bodies. Like pregnancy, breastfeeding is exclusively women's burden and benefit. In fact, distinguishing discrimination against breastfeeding from that against pregnancy may be splitting hairs—for many women breastfeeding is a natural extension of pregnancy." If this link can be made legally, the PDA would offer protection to breastfeeding women at work.

In an article entitled "Out of the Mouths of Babies: No Mother's Milk for U.S. Children" (*Hamline Law Review,* Winter, 1995), author Isabelle Schallreuter Olson points out how it is logical to consider breastfeeding as a "related medical condition" under the PDA. In effect, she says federal laws give more protection to the three-month-old fetus requiring the mother to be on bedrest than a three-month-old child requiring a mother's breastmilk. Olson says that women seeking protection or redress using the PDA need to argue the medical benefits of breastfeeding.

The Equal Employment Opportunity Act of 1972

This amendment was created to enforce Title VII, and from it Congress created the Equal Employment Opportunity Commission (EEOC). The EEOC has the authority to file suit in Federal District Court on behalf of individuals who allege discrimination. Further explanation of the EEOC is included in the next section, "How to File a Discrimination Suit."

The Constitution of the United States

In the case of Janice Dike (described earlier), the Ninth and Fourteenth Amendments were used as the basis for the litigation. That case established a precedent that breastfeeding is an activity protected by the Constitution, and as such, the state cannot encroach on that right without very compelling reasons. Building a case based on violation of your constitutional rights is another avenue you can travel when alleging unfair employer practices. Some experts suggest that if you are a public employee, the constitutional route may be your best strategy, while the Title VII route is best for employees of private corporations.

The Ninth Amendment to the Constitution states:

"The enumeration in the Constitution, of certain rights, shall not be construed to deny or disparage others retained by the people." [This means that Congress

cannot adopt laws that infringe on a person's fundamental liberties.]

The Ninth Amendment issue in the Dike case was that the
school violated Ms. Dike's right to privacy by interfering with
her freedom of personal choice in a matter pertaining to family life.

Section 1 of the Fourteenth Amendment to the Constitution states:

> "All persons born or naturalized in the United States,
> and subject to the jurisdiction thereof, are citizens of
> the United States and of the state wherein they reside.
> No state shall make or enforce any law which shall
> abridge the privileges or immunities of citizens of the
> United States; nor shall any state deprive any person of
> life, liberty, or property, without due process of law;
> nor deny to any person within its jurisdiction the
> equal rights or equal protection of the laws." [States
> cannot deny equal rights or equal protection to any
> person.]

The Fourteenth Amendment issue in the Dike case was
that the school violated the Fourteenth Amendment's guarantee of due process by interfering with her liberty as a parent
to direct the upbringing of her child.

In her article, Isabelle Schallreuter Olson expresses a
rather dim view of the constitutional arguments for breastfeeding, in spite of the precedent set in the *Dike* case. Against
the state's compelling interest, Olson says, "the right to breastfeed stands little chance." Institutions can always argue, as the
school system did in *Dike,* that the breastfeeding interferes
with the safe or smooth operation of the system. "As a constitutional right, it is no more than a fancy plaque on the wall because it neither protects a woman's right to breastfeed nor
does it encourage employers . . . to accommodate breastfeeding women."

The Family and Medical Leave Act

In August 1993, after a nine-year battle, the Family and Medical Leave Act (FMLA) was signed into law. The FMLA gives those who work for companies with fifty or more employees the right to take up to twelve weeks of unpaid leave a year to care for a newborn or newly adopted child, a seriously ill family member, or to recover from a serious health condition, including pregnancy. Since the law was enacted, about two-thirds of the businesses covered by the act have complied and changed their leave policies, according to the Women's Legal Defense Fund, which proposed the first bill over a decade ago. The current law is a much less generous version of the original bill, and the Defense Fund points out that fewer than half of American employees and less than 11 percent of American businesses are covered by the new law. But it's a start.

To qualify, your employer must have fifty or more employees on the payroll for twenty work weeks during the current or preceding year, fifty employees must work within seventy-five miles of your worksite, and you must have worked for your employer for at least twelve months and for at least 1,250 hours during the last year.

If you qualify for the leave, the law entitles you to twelve weeks off per twelve-month period. This leave can be taken intermittently—days or weeks or even hours at a time. When you return, your employer must give you either the same job you had when you left or a position with equivalent benefits, pay, working conditions, and security. When you have a baby, your spouse is also entitled to his own twelve weeks of leave. While you are on leave, your employer must continue to pay your health insurance coverage. Other benefits can be discontinued, but when you return, those benefits must be returned to you without your having to re-apply.

There are other specific ramifications and entitlements under this law, and you might want to familiarize yourself with them fully before you apply for leave. For this, we recommend the Women's Legal Defense Fund's Guide to the Family and Medical Leave Act, which you can get by sending $8 to Family and Medical Leave Act Materials, The Women's Legal Defense Fund, 1875 Connecticut Avenue NW, #710, Washington, D.C. 20009. More information about enforcement of the FMLA is available through the U.S. Department of Labor, Wage and Hour Division, 200 Constitution Avenue NW, Washington, D.C. 20210, (202) 219-8305.

If your employer denies your request for family or medical leave, you can file a complaint by contacting the regional office of the U.S. Department of Labor, Wage and Hour Division. If the problem cannot be resolved, the labor department may investigate further and can sue your employer on your behalf. You might also wish to hire an attorney who specializes in employee rights. If the labor department does not file a suit on your behalf, you can file your own lawsuit in state or federal court. One such suit was brought by Kevin Knussman, a Maryland state trooper who was denied family leave after the birth of his daughter. His employer told him, erroneously, that the leave policy only applied to the primary caregiver of the child, and when Knussman said that because of his wife's illness he was the primary caregiver, he was told that the law only applied to women.

Despite a lot of whining by naysayers during the passage of this law, recent research has shown the Family and Medical Leave Act has had a positive impact on employee morale and loyalty. The First Chicago Corporation, the nation's tenth largest bank holding company, found that employees who were guaranteed family and medical leave are more productive and more committed to the company.

NEGOTIATE FIRST

Discrimination suits are time-consuming and costly. They require extensive documentation, evidence, and testimony, and the personal price can be high. Before you commit both your resources and your precious emotional energy, you should exhaust all other means of conciliation with your employer. Hopefully, a complete knowledge of your rights and of the legal precedents that might apply in your case will give you the confidence and the backing to negotiate with your employer and come to an agreement without needing to pull out the big guns.

Before you approach your employer with the working/breastfeeding strategy you have devised, make sure it is well organized. Prepare written notes in which you have outlined how you plan to meet your job obligations while you are breastfeeding. Anticipate what your employer's concerns might be and have responses and contingency suggestions ready.

There is no reason to feel apologetic about your wish to breastfeed your baby. Remember, what you want to do is not inappropriate, nor is it unreasonable. Approach your discussions with your employer with the confidence that your job and your parenting are compatible. If your plan includes a reduction in your work load for a while, for example through a reassignment or a switch to part-time work, realize that this is a temporary and not an extraordinary request.

Know your company's policies on maternity leave, flexible scheduling, and part-time work. Read your employee's manual, and talk with other women who have had babies, particularly those who have breastfed. However, don't assume that you are limited to what women before you have done. Decide what *you* need and ask for it.

Many employers are reticent about flexible scheduling or part-time arrangements that accommodate child care. They are afraid to set precedents. You will need to demonstrate how your job and your breastfeeding can be blended. You are not asking for concessions; rather, you are a conscientious employee presenting an arrangement that is different but entirely workable. As for setting precedents, that's the whole point, isn't it?

Write a description of your job, detailing the responsibilities and how you expect to fulfill them. This exercise gives you a chance to demonstrate, both to yourself and your employer, the extent of your experience, contribution, and importance to the company. Mention how you exceeded production quota last month, the big ad campaign you organized, or the excellent job evaluation you received at the last salary review.

While you are out on maternity leave, stay in touch with your employer and coworkers. Call or get together for lunch. Keep up to date about what is going on in your industry or profession.

If your workplace or employer continues to thwart your effort to work and breastfeed, follow your company's policies for filing a formal grievance. If you are a member of a union, find out the procedure for filing a grievance through the union. Keep a diary, in your own handwriting, of dates, conversations, and actions relevant to your discrimination claim.

After exhausting these internal remedies, a legal route may be your only means toward conciliation with your employer. Knowledge of the cases described in the previous section may help you to convince a recalcitrant employer that your complaint is justified, and thus divert a full-fledged court battle.

Finally, keep records of everything you have done in a conscientious effort to come to an agreement with your employer. If and when you get to court it will be significant in showing that you acted responsibly and that you considered the requirements of your job at all times.

HOW TO BRING A DISCRIMINATION SUIT

At this point, Title VII is the most widely used law in discrimination litigation. To bring a Title VII lawsuit in district court, you must first file a formal complaint with the Equal Employment Opportunity Commission (EEOC). This must be done within 180 days after the alleged act of discrimination. In states where there are local Fair Employment Practices Agencies you have up to 240 days, and in some cases up to 300 days to file your complaint. However, it is best to act within the 180-day limit to make sure you don't lose your chance to bring a suit.

The EEOC is a structured agency with forty-eight field offices located throughout the country. In most areas you can find the number of your field office in the telephone directory under "U.S. Government, Equal Employment Opportunity Commission." The address of the national headquarters is listed at the end of this chapter. If you are thinking about retaining a private attorney and bringing your own suit without the intervention of the EEOC, you should still have a complaint on record with the EEOC within the 180-day limit.

When you call the EEOC, ask for the "intake unit." Personnel in the intake unit handle inquiries and gather the information about your allegation of discrimination. The information elicited during the intake interview will be used to develop your formal charge of discrimination. You will then come to the office to swear the charge under oath, or you can do this by mail. The intake officer may try to discourage you from filing the charge. But by law the EEOC must take your charge if you insist that it be filed.

You can file a charge as an individual or you can file on behalf of a group of employees who have experienced the same type of discrimination. This latter charge is called a class action suit (the discriminatory act involves a whole class of employees) and is a way to benefit a number of women as a result of your particular action.

Also, organizations such as civil rights groups, women's organizations, or labor unions can file a lawsuit on your behalf. For example, in the case of Janice Dike, the suit was brought by the Florida Teaching Profession—National Education Association.

Once the charge has been filed, the EEOC will then notify the employer. If your employer reacts by firing, reassigning, demoting, or harassing you, you are entitled to claim retaliation and ask for EEOC intervention immediately.

The EEOC is required to defer your charge for sixty days

to a state or local agency, if there is one, before it assumes jurisdiction over your case. States vary in how this is handled, so be sure you understand the procedure in your state. Ask who will have jurisdiction over your case.

If you are a federal employee, the procedure is somewhat different, and you should consult the EEOC for the steps to follow in your situation.

Next, the EEOC will act as mediator in an agreement between you and your employer. A fact-finding conference may be held to define and explore the issues and hopefully to reach a resolution. If the employer offers relief from the discrimination, such as job reinstatement or salary compensation, it will be up to you to decide whether to accept those terms. In the case of a breastfeeding issue, the employer may agree to your plan but do nothing for other women who may follow in your footsteps. You will need to decide how broad you want the final resolution to be. If you hope to make some sweeping changes in the policies with regard to mothers and child care, you will need to take this into consideration when deciding whether to accept an offer that benefits you alone. On the other hand, the time and money involved in continuing with a lawsuit must also be taken into consideration. You may wish to retain an attorney before the fact-finding conference to advise you about the terms that are offered.

If there is no resolution at the fact-finding conference and the EEOC finds cause, the EEOC will either continue to investigate your case or issue you a right-to-sue in district court. You are free to sue without an EEOC right-to-sue notice at any time, but it may be harder to get an attorney to take your case. You can also request a notice of right-to-sue to bring your own lawsuit before the EEOC investigation (to shorten the time it often takes for the EEOC process to be complete), but because of deadlines, you should have an attorney before you make this request.

Remedies available under Title VII include requiring an employer to end the discriminatory practices, reinstatement, promotion, transfer, awarding of back pay and benefits (including fringe benefits, overtime, leave and vacation pay, retirement contributions), restoration of seniority, and new policies of affirmative actions to end discrimination of women in that workplace.

Whether you base your lawsuit on Title VII or on constitutional principles will depend on your particular circumstances and the advice of your legal counsel. It is possible that your attorney will file charges on both grounds. You can assist your attorney, and thus reduce your fees, by your familiarity with the cases described in the previous section (pages 176–85). The notations following the names of the suits are called the "cite," which is the reference number for the case record.

File Your Complaint with the EEOC Within 180 Days After the Discriminatory Treatment.

HOW TO FIND AN ATTORNEY

Under Title VII, your attorney's fees will be paid by the party you are suing—but only if you win. This means that the stronger your case, the better chance you have of finding an attorney to take it. While you may have to pay a fee up front, along with expenses as you go along, these costs can be reimbursed with the money awarded by the court. If you win your suit, you do not have to pay any attorney's fees out of your own personal earnings from the lawsuit.

Besides a lawyer or firm willing to tackle a costly endeavor such as discrimination, you need legal expertise in civil-rights litigation, itself a complex specialty. Sometimes a woman is able to rally financial assistance from organizations or groups of individuals who raise money on her behalf. There are few working women (or anyone for that matter) who can afford to dip into their own pockets to finance such a lawsuit. However, if you have a strong case, it will be worth all the effort it takes to find an attorney or firm who will take your case on its merits.

You will need to target an attorney who is creative and has expertise in civil-rights issues. Here are some suggestions for finding one:

- Word of mouth.
- A lawyer you know. (Ask specifically, What is your experience in civil-rights litigation?)
- Referral from a lawyer you know and trust.
- Ask the EEOC for its lawyer referral list.
- Contact the Fair Employment Practices office, and your local women's or civil rights organization (NOW, League of Women Voters, La Leche League).
- Check with the state bar association, and ask for the Labor & Employment Law section. Most of these practitioners represent employers, but they will refer you.
- Go to the clerk's office in your courthouse, and ask for names of attorneys who have filed recent civil-rights litigation.
- Contact resources at the end of this chapter.

STAND UP FOR YOUR RIGHTS

Although it is popular for politicians and lawmakers to applaud motherhood, apple pie, and breastfeeding, actual laws and policies to provide real support for breastfeeding women in the workplace do not match the rhetoric. As we've shown in this chapter, there are legal arguments to protect breastfeeding women in the workplace, but few have been codified into case law or civil-rights law.

In her article, Olson points out that the average woman will spend about two-thirds of her life with no children under the age of eighteen. Contrast to that the amount of time that most women will spend breastfeeding exclusively—perhaps six months—and we are not looking at a huge interruption in anyone's work life. It is absurd to think that giving a woman support for a few months of breastfeeding, even a year, will halt the wheels of commerce. On the contrary, the economic benefits of breastfeeding certainly outweigh the costs, with healthier babies costing less in insurance payments for illness, and female employees who are loyal and happy.

Stand up for what you want, says Patricia Lee, the attorney for Judy Deeley, whose story appeared at the beginning of this chapter. Lee says that when she receives calls from breastfeeding women who are having difficulty in their workplaces, she advises them of their rights and encourages them to make these rights clearly known to their employers. Most often, when a woman stands up for herself, employers go along with the woman's request. What company wants to be hauled through the press and perhaps the courts because it wasn't nice to a breastfeeding mother? From a public relations standpoint, this is not smart. Lee says: "When it's put in the right light and pursued aggressively, they will back down."

WHERE TO TURN FOR HELP

Catalyst, 14 E. 60th Street, New York, NY 10022

Child Care Law Center, 625 Market Street, Suite 815, San Francisco, CA 94105

Coal Employment Project, 16221 Sunny Knoll Court, Dumfries, VA 22026

Equal Employment Opportunity Commission, local office, or national headquarters at: 2401 E Street NW, Washington, D.C. 20506

International Labor Organization Staff Union, 4, route des Morillons, CH-1211 Geneva 22, Switzerland

International Lactation Consultants Association (ILCA), P.O. Box 4031, University of Virginia Station, Charlottesville, VA 22903

La Leche League International, local chapter, or headquarters at: 9616 Minneapolis Avenue, Franklin Park, IL 60131 (ask for the "Breastfeeding Rights Packet")

League of Women Voters, local chapter, or national headquarters at: 1730 M Street NW, Washington, D.C. 20036

National Commission on Working Women, 2000 P Street NW, Suite 508, Washington, D.C. 20036

NOW (National Organization of Women), local chapter, or national headquarters at: P.O. Box 37002, Washington, D.C. 20013

National Women's Law Center, 1751 N Street NW, Washington, D.C. 20036

National Women's Political Caucus, 1275 K Street NW, Suite 750, Washington, D.C. 20005

Wider Opportunities for Women, 1325 G Street NW, Washington, D.C. 20005

Working Women (National Organization of Office Workers), Legal Support Office, 16221 Sunny Knoll Lane, Dumfries, VA 22026

Women's Legal Defense Fund, 2000 P Street NW, Suite 400, Washington, D.C. 20036

Resources

GOOD BOOKS ABOUT BREASTFEEDING

The Breastfeeding Answer Book. N. Mohrbacher and J. Stock (La Leche League International, 1991).

Breastfeeding Product Guide. Frantz, Kittie (Geddes Productions, 1994).

Breastfeeding Your Baby. Carl Jones (Macmillan, 1993).

Breastfeeding Your Baby. Sheila Kitzinger (Alfred A. Knopf, 1989).

The Complete Book of Breastfeeding. Marvin Eiger and Sally Wendkos Olds (Workman, 1987).

Eat Well, Lose Weight While Breastfeeding. Eileen Behan, R.D. (Villard Books, 1992).

Motherwear, Inc. A free forty-page catalog with clothing and products designed for the breastfeeding mother. Contact Ms. Jharna Morrisey, Public Relations, 320 Riverside Drive, Northampton, MA 01060; (413) 586-1978, Fax (413) 586-2712, e-mail: jharna@crocker.com

The Nursing Mother's Companion. Kathleen Huggins (The Harvard Common Press, 1990).

Nutrition During Lactation. Institute of Medicine (The National Academy Press, 1991).

Successful Breastfeeding: A Practical Guide for Mothers and Mid- wives and Others Supporting Breastfeeding Mothers. Royal College of Midwives Staff (Churchill Livingstone, 1991).

What to Expect The First Year. Eisenberg, Murkoff, and Hathaway (Workman, 1989).

What to Expect The Toddler Years. Eisenberg, Murkoff, and Hath- away (Workman, 1994).

What to Expect When You're Expecting. Eisenberg, Murkoff, and Hathaway (Workman, 1984).

Womanly Art of Breastfeeding. 5th rev. ed. (La Leche League Inter- national, 1991).

Working and Caring. T. Berry Brazelton (Addison-Wesley, 1985).

The Working Parents' Survival Guide. Sally Wendkos Olds (Bantam Books, 1983).

The following books are directed to health professionals. Though the material is more technical, they are excellent resources, if you can find them in your local library.

Breastfeeding: A Guide For the Medical Profession, Fourth Edition. Ruth A. Lawrence (Mosby, 1994).

Breastfeeding and Human Lactation. Kathleen Auerbach and Jan Riordan (Jones and Bartlett, 1993).

Breastfeeding Resource Handbook for the HealthCare Professional. San Diego County Breastfeeding Coalition, c/o Children's Hospital and Health Center, 3020 Children's Way MC 5058, San Diego, CA 92123-4282.

BREASTFEEDING SUPPORT ORGANIZATIONS

Geddes Productions, 10546 McVine Avenue, Sunland, CA 91040, telephone: (818) 951-2809. Kittie Frantz video series, Dr. Righard's self-attachment video, slides, flip charts, poster teach- ing cards, patient tear-off handouts, overheads, and photo blowups are available.

Health Education Associates, 8 Sebastian Way #13, Sandwich, MA 02563. Publishes a number of informative pamphlets on breastfeeding, as well as other adult and child health care topics.

Human Lactation Center, 666 Sturges Highway, Westport, CT 06880, telephone: (203) 259-5995, Fax: (203) 259-7667. Conducts research, encourages breastfeeding.

Human Milk Banking Association of North America, Inc., P.O. Box 370464, West Hartford, CT 06137-0464.

International Childbirth Education Association (ICEA), P.O. Box 20048, Minneapolis, MN 55420, telephone: (612) 854-8660.

International Lactation Consultant Association, 201 Brown Avenue, Evanston, IL 60202, telephone: (708) 665-6848. A network of lactation consultants (persons who advise and support nursing mothers) focusing on research and scientific articles relating to the support of breastfeeding.

The Lactation Institute, 16161 Ventura Boulevard, Suite 223, Encion, CA 91436, telephone: (818) 995-1913.

La Leche League International, 1400 North Meachum Road, Schaumburg, IL 60173-4826, telephone: (847) 519-7730, Fax: (708) 519-0035. A vast breastfeeding support and resource network, with thousands of local chapters. You can contact the above address, or consult your local directory for a chapter in your town.

National Alliance for Breastfeeding Advocacy, Office of Educational Services, 254 Conant Road, Weston, MA 02193, telephone: (617) 893-3553. Formed to help protect, support, and promote breastfeeding, the Alliance takes political action and provides educational resources for breastfeeding mothers.

National Association of Child Care Resource and Referral Agencies, 1319 F Street NW, Suite #810, Washington D.C. 20004, telephone: (202) 393-5501, e-mail HN5018@Handsnet.org.

Nursing Mothers Counsel, P.O. Box 50063, Palo Alto, CA 94303-0063, telephone: (415) 599-3669.

WIC (Women and Infant Children) Program. A supplemental food program for pregnant and nursing women, infants, and children who are unable to meet their special nutritional needs. You can locate your local WIC office by calling the city or county health department.

ADDITIONAL RESOURCES

Families and Work Institute, 330 7th Avenue, 14th Floor, New York, NY 10001 (212) 465-2044. Provides direction on how to balance family and work.

Healthy Mothers, Healthy Babies National Coalition, 409 12th Street SW, Room 253, Washington D.C. 20024-2188, (202) 863-2458. Provides health education for pregnant women and families.

National Association of Working Women, Survival Hotline (800) 522-0925. Offers counseling on workers' rights, harassment.

VIDEO RESOURCES

The Art of Successful Breastfeeding, Dr. Verity Livingstone; to order call 1-800-667-1500.

Breastfeeding Techniques that Work™, Volume 5, "Successful Working Mothers," Kittie Frantz, Geddes Productions, 10546 McVine, Sunland, CA 91040. (818) 951-2809. http://www.geddespro.com

COMPUTER RESOURCES

America Online, CompuServe, Prodigy and other on-line services offer bulletin boards, chat rooms, and the ability to search the internet for breastfeeding information. Bulletin boards allow you to post questions on a specific topic. Individuals from around the world may respond. Chat rooms provide an excellent opportunity to interact with working breastfeeding mothers from all across the country. These three major services and many other local internet access providers offer an unlimited and ever-changing breastfeeding information base.

All on-line companies provide support services that can assist you in locating appropriate bulletin boards and chat lines.

There are thousands of breastfeeding-related sites to be discovered simply through searching—or surfing—the Net.

America Online	800-827-6364
CompuServe	800-848-8990
Prodigy	800-776-3449

Index

You can obtain additional copies of this book at your local bookseller, or by using the coupon below.

ORDER FORM

Please send me

_____ copies of *Breastfeeding and the Working Mother,*
       revised edition @ $11.95 per copy
       ISBN 0-312-15486-0

Enclosed is a check or money order, payable to Publishers Book & Audio, in the amount of $ _____ (please include shipping and handling charges of $3.00 for the first book, and $1.00 for each additional book).

Send books to: Name _____

                     Address _____

                               _____

                               _____

Send this coupon and your payment to: Publishers Book & Audio, P.O. Box 070059, Staten Island, NY 10307. Please allow four to six weeks for delivery.

    For bulk orders (10 or more copies), contact St. Martin's Press, Special Markets Division, 175 Fifth Avenue, New York, NY 10010. Or call, toll free, 1-800-221-7945, extension #645, 636, 628, or 662.